FODMAP DIET

The Beginner's Guide to Managing Digestive Disorders

Jan Ellenberger

© **Copyright 2020 - All rights reserved.**

The content contained within this book may not be reproduced, duplicated or transmitted without direct written permission from the author or the publisher.

Under no circumstances will any blame or legal responsibility be held against the publisher, or author, for any damages, reparation, or monetary loss due to the information contained within this book, either directly or indirectly.

Legal Notice:

This book is copyright protected. It is only for personal use. You cannot amend, distribute, sell, use, quote or paraphrase any part, or the content within this book, without the consent of the author or publisher.

Disclaimer Notice:

Please note the information contained within this document is for educational and entertainment purposes only. All effort has been executed to present accurate, up to date, reliable, complete information. No warranties of any kind are declared or implied. Readers acknowledge that the author is not engaged in the rendering of legal, financial, medical or professional advice. The content within this book has been derived from various sources. Please consult a licensed professional before attempting any techniques outlined in this book.

By reading this document, the reader agrees that under no circumstances is the author responsible for any losses, direct or indirect, that are incurred as a result of the use of the information contained within this document, including, but not limited to, errors, omissions, or inaccuracies.

Table of Contents

INTRODUCTION 1

CHAPTER 1: MEET YOUR GUT 11

CHAPTER 2: MICROBIOME - AN ARMY OF MICROBES KEEPING YOU HEALTHY 23

CHAPTER 3: WHAT IS YOUR GUT TELLING YOU? 41

CHAPTER 4: IS YOUR GUT LEAKING? 79

CHAPTER 5: IS FODMAP DIET THE ANSWER? 99

CHAPTER 6: FODMAP DIET CHART 117

CHAPTER 7: THREE PHASES OF THE FODMAP DIET 143

CHAPTER 8: LOW-FODMAP DIET BREAKFASTS 165

CHAPTER 9: LOW-FODMAP DIET MAIN MEALS 181

CHAPTER 10: LOW-FODMAP DIET DESSERTS 201

CHAPTER 11: LOW-FODMAP DIET SNACKS 217

CONCLUSION 231

REFERENCE LIST 235

Introduction

"You are what you eat." This adage has proven to be true since our body construct and functionality is composed of the nutrients we ingest, digest, and assimilate. It's the ability, or inability to effectively digest and process certain foods that will make all the difference in our health, comfort, and overall well-being, so we need to be sure our diets are optimal for us, and don't have adverse effects. We want to feel our best, free from discomfort or debilitating conditions. Some dietary problems can extend beyond the gut to other parts of the body, including the immune system, and lead to the onset of other, more serious issues down the line.

With so many dietary disorders prevalent today, many people have become dependent on a variety of supplements, and medications, some of which have side effects that result in more medicine. While many disorders and diseases require professional medical attention, in many cases, dietary modification can play an important role in reducing or eliminating digestive disorders.

This book will introduce you to the FODMAP diet, which was developed in collaboration with universities in London, England, and Australia. It's more than another diet for you to consider; rather, it is a system of identifying virtually every type of food that may trigger a disorder, disease, or other negative condition. But rather than stopping there, the FODMAP diet guides you through a process of elimination, followed by gradual reintroduction of various foods, so you don't have to eliminate many foods to root out a few that are not right for you.

Before we get to the details of how to effectively use the FODMAP diet, I want to build your knowledge of how the digestive system works, from the fundamentals of how food is digested and turned into the key nutrients your body needs, to the beneficial microbiota, which are the trillions of beneficial bacteria in our gut. We'll cover the many gastrointestinal disorders and diseases that can not only cause discomfort and inconvenience, but can lead to chronic, or long lasting disorders. There's a chapter dedicated to one specific chronic digestive disorder, called leaky gut, which is not yet fully understood, but many medical authorities believe is triggered by diet. We will also cover the FODMAP diet, and how to cook in this style to enjoy a plethora of delicious food options.

Overview

This is meant to familiarize you with the fundamentals of your digestive system, the microbiome, common digestive system disorders, leaky gut, and the concept of the FODMAP diet.

Your Digestive System

You will meet your gut and discover the surprisingly elaborate, yet highly functional gastrointestinal tract, and the organs and bacteria that support its function. The digestive process begins as soon as you take a bite and start to chew. When solid food enters your mouth, it undergoes a cycle of grinding by your molars, and moistening by saliva, a process which also begins to break down the carbohydrates in the food. After you swallow and as the food passes down your esophagus and into your stomach, it encounters a barrage of breaking down procedures by enzymes, bacteria, and strong gastric acids, as well as more grinding, until the food has been reduced to a concentrated paste of nutrients.

The original food has been reduced to the carbohydrates, proteins, and fats that are essential for life, and are now in a simplified form of simple sugars, amino acids, and fatty acids, as they begin their passage through the small intestine, where the digestive enzymes and bacteria continue to reduce the food to the form your body can absorb. It's from here that the nutrients pass through the intestinal walls to enter the bloodstream, and reach and sustain every cell, every organ, and every muscle. The digestive process is further supported by the pancreas, liver, and gallbladder. The remaining food and water continue into and through the large intestine, on its way to elimination.

By now you will have noticed that bacteria have a role in digestion. Certain bacteria participate in the breaking down of food for digestion, but more recent studies show the greater presence and diverse role of beneficial bacteria throughout the gastrointestinal tract—the microbiome.

The Microbiome

> *"Everyday we live and every meal we eat influences the great microbial organ inside us - for better or for worse."*
> *- Giulia Enders*

Dr. Giulia Enders, a published author and medical practitioner from Germany has inspired much of what we now know about this emerging science. She is credited as a pioneer of the concept that trillions of bacteria live in our gut and substantially influence our digestion and the overall health and stability of our immune system. At the time, when Enders began her presentations, few if any medical and dietary professionals even knew what we now recognize as the microbiome, and its diverse, influential role in maintaining our health.

Now, it's generally recognized that our guts are host to this vast population of innumerable types of bacteria, as well fungi, and (mostly) beneficial viruses, as well as parasites. The term "microbiota" refers to a vast population of microscopic organisms, and "microbiome" is the network that extends through the digestive system to influence the organs, the central nervous system, and the immune system.

You will see later how the microbiota affect your body weight, cardiovascular health, mental health, and allergies, as well as your immune system's functions. It can trigger autoimmune conditions, including chronic inflammation, and diseases like rheumatoid arthritis, diabetes, and may even contribute to the onset of cancer.

Numerous prebiotics and probiotics are available today; these nutrients have been developed to nurture existing microbiota, and to introduce new strains of living beneficial bacteria into the gut. We'll cover the sources and potential values of these types of dietary supplements, as part of your own dietary practices.

Digestive Disorders

Do you suffer from digestive disorders? More than 60 million Americans experience acid reflux at least once a month, when stomach acid leaks up into the esophagus, and gives us that painful burning sensation we call heartburn. When the backwash that causes acid reflux and heartburn becomes chronic, or continues, it's considered gastroesophageal reflux disease (GERD), and requires treatment to prevent irritation of the lining of the esophagus. Although acid reflux is believed to occur from relaxation of the gastroesophageal sphincter, which normally prevents stomach contents from leaking out, a diet targeted to your specific personal needs may reduce the symptoms of GERD.

Another gastric disorder, IBS, or irritable bowel syndrome, affects the large intestine, and causes cramping, gas, diarrhea, bloating, constipation, and abdominal pain. It tends to be a chronic, long term condition, but as with treating GERD, it can be managed in many cases by controlling diet and lifestyle.

Leaky Gut

Leaky gut syndrome is a more recently diagnosed disorder, and while it has not yet been officially recognized, many gastrology specialists are taking it seriously. It affects the intestinal lining, and may result from gaps, or openings, in the walls of the intestines, which enable toxins and bacteria to enter the bloodstream. These gaps are the usually smaller openings that let digested nutrients through to the bloodstream, but inflammation caused by autoimmune responses may cause these small gaps to open wider, creating intestinal permeability and permitting the leakages.

Recent studies suggest that leaky gut may be the cause of IBD, or inflammatory bowel disease, and also may be a precursor to type 1 diabetes. Leaky gut shares many of the symptoms of IBS, IBD, Crohn's disease and other disorders, making it hard to diagnose. More studies are underway, but fortunately it is a condition that may be treated through dietary modifications: this is where the FODMAP diet comes into play..

The FODMAP Diet

At this point, you should be ready to plunge into the FODMAP diet and the identification of fermentable oligosaccharides, disaccharides, monosaccharides, and polyps, and what this all means for you. In simplest terms, these are carbohydrates that resist normal digestion, and cause disruption in the gut, especially among the microbiota. The FODMAP diet is frequently the go-to solution for many intestinal disorders, including leaky gut.

Subsequently, we'll go through the extensive lists of foods that the FODMAP diet allows, tolerates, or restricts, so you can easily understand what can stay, and what must go, at least initially. There are three phases in the FODMAP diet:

1. The initial elimination phase.
2. The gradual reintroduction phase.
3. The final integration phase.

We will cover all three phases, with advice on how to get through the most restrictive first phase, known as the elimination phase. You will need to stay in this restrictive phase until the symptoms of your gastrointestinal disorder are gone. This will prove it's "something" in your diet; you just won't know yet which foods are causing the disorder. The second, or reintroduction phase is where you will gradually bring selected restricted foods back into your diet, to give them a trial to see whether or not symptoms return. The third, or integration phase, is when your diet has been cleaned out of disruptive foods, and you are now free to eat everything that was reintroduced without returning symptoms.

The remaining chapters are devoted to helping you enjoy all three phases of the FODMAP diet by providing delicious recipes and ideas to make your meals as satisfying as they are healthy. You'll be given the recipe-constructing basics, so you can create your own specialties, and include the foods you like, while staying within the FODMAP guidelines.

Before we begin I want to introduce my qualifications by explaining how nutrition and digestive health are my passion, and how I can help you, as I have helped so many others before you. I am a dietitian who specializes in digestive disorders, and excited to share my advanced knowledge within these pages. I have learned through many years of professional experience with patients, research studies, and nutritional experiments, how impactful digestive problems can be on your quality of life. There are an increasing number of digestive diseases and conditions that are being diagnosed as more is learned about the complexity of the gastrointestinal tract, and the organs and systems that support it.

Fortunately, science and medicine have made considerable progress in understanding these disorders, and in developing effective treatments to relieve and prevent the symptoms. I am especially optimistic about the good results coming from the FODMAP diet, which enables you to identify the specific foods that are giving you trouble, without forcing you to surrender many of the foods you love.

Most people do not understand nutrition, and the importance of maintaining good gut health and balance, especially where the microbiome is concerned. They are astonished to learn that an army of trillions of bacteria and other microbes live within us, and contribute to our digestive and overall health. As I will show you, the microbiome can become your best friend and ally in maintaining a healthy digestive system.

I have written this book to help you understand nutrition and digestion, and to learn how to make the right nutritional choices, and stop making the wrong choices that can lead to chronic illnesses. This book is dedicated to you, and to your health, well-being and fullness of life.

Chapter 1:

Meet Your Gut

What we commonly call the gut is your gastrointestinal digestive system. This chapter will introduce you to what the gut is, what its component organs are, and how it works to accomplish the complex process of digesting food and putting its nutrients to work for you. The digestive system is busy 24/7, contributing to the ongoing process of rebuilding and repairing cells, enabling growth, and providing energy. It's an amazing, highly efficient process that has evolved and kept our species and most vertebrates alive and well for countless millennia, and is critical today to your well-being and health.

The Sequence of Digestion

The digestive system is elaborate and performs a wide range of functions, but the effectiveness of each person's digestive system can vary based on factors ranging from genetics to illnesses and the physical condition. When necessary, alternative diets can help an individual to feel healthier. Among the many diets that exist and you have probably heard about, the FODMAP diet is uniquely capable of helping evaluate and identify a person's optimal diet, through the identification of foods that may be risky, and need to be eliminated from the diet. We'll plunge deeply into the FODMAP diet in subsequent chapters, but here is an overview of the system that your diet directly influences.

Your digestive system consists of the gastrointestinal (GI) tract and the closely involved pancreas, liver and gallbladder. The digestion of everything you eat begins at your mouth, continues down through the esophagus, enters the stomach, and is further processed by the small intestine, where the pancreas, liver, and gallbladder are involved, then on to the large intestine, or colon, and eventually, the food is deposited in the rectum, and subsequently exits.

Let's take a step-by-step tour through the entire digestive process.

The Mouth

Considering that all food enters our bodies through the mouth, it's the appropriate place for the digestive process to begin. You may not envision the mouth as a digestive organ, but the action does indeed start here. What do you first do to solid food that you put in your mouth? You chew it in a process that breaks the food into small pieces or a soft paste, which we designate as step one in the digestive process. Our teeth evolved to molars that are perfectly designed to crush and pulverize the food so that it's ready for the next step, which is the effect of saliva, produced by the salivary glands. Saliva serves two purposes: to moisten the food and begin the enzymatic process of breaking down the starch in the food into smaller pieces. This first step of enzymes in the saliva when breaking down food is minimal compared to what will happen in the stomach, but it's a start. Digestion is now underway, and you haven't even swallowed yet!

Once you swallow, which is a reflex that is helped by the action of your tongue pushing the food into your throat, and which is done mostly automatically when your brain receives a message that the food in your mouth is sufficiently ground up and moistened. The food passes briefly through your throat or pharynx and enters the esophagus. But just before the food descends into the esophagus, the epiglottis, a small but important flap of muscle, automatically closes over the windpipe entry, so the food continues into the esophagus and not into the lungs.

The Esophagus

This is a tube-shaped flexible structure that transports the food from the throat, down through the chest, through the lower esophageal sphincter, and into the stomach. The sphincter lets descending food pass through and tightens to prevent food and stomach acids from rising back up into the esophagus, where it can irritate and cause acid reflux and other gastroesophageal disorders.

While gravity plays a key role in helping food to descend the length of the esophagus, a series of contractions called peristalsis is also present. As you will see, peristalsis plays an important role throughout the digestive process.

What is peristalsis? Food moves through the GI tract thanks to the layer of muscles that surround the hollow tract and provide the power of peristalsis needed to push the food down through the tract. In addition to pushing solids and liquids through the tract, the squeezing, contracting motion mixes the digestive material, adding to its breakdown for eventual digestion and assimilation. The cycle of peristalsis is activated by a muscle contracting behind the food mass, and a muscle in front of the food that relaxes to let the food continue its forward motion. Imagine a continuous squeezing, relaxing, squeezing, relaxing cycle that keeps food moving on its path.

The Stomach

This is where the digestive process kicks into high gear. Food that enters the sac-like stomach is immediately subjected to a dual process of grinding, under pressure from the muscles that surround the stomach, and the chemical action of the digestive juices, which contain enzymes, proteins that trigger chemical reactions, and hydrochloric acid that is excreted into the stomach. Added to the digestive process are the actions of beneficial bacteria, as part of the microbiome (which we'll cover in the next chapter).

Depending on the type of food being processed, its passage through the stomach may vary: proteins, for example, digest more slowly than carbohydrates, which break into simple sugars, and fats, which in turn further break into fatty acids. Proteins, in contrast, are made of more complex molecules called peptides, which need to be broken down into simpler amino acids, the building blocks of proteins. In all cases, when food leaves the stomach to enter the small intestine, it is the consistency of a paste, composed of partially digested food and digestive juices, and is called chyme.

Small Intestine

As food enters the small intestine, its passage is again aided by peristalsis, and the digestive process continues, as enzymes from the liver and pancreas go to work. The small intestine is coiled up in the abdomen but would be up to 20 feet long if fully extended.

The small intestine is composed of three sections. Food first passes through the duodenum, where the breaking down and digestion of food particles continues. Bacteria make some of the digestive enzymes, especially to break down complex carbohydrates, including starches. The food continues through the second section, the jejunum, and then into the ileum, where the digested nutrients of the food and water cross the intestinal lining and pass through the walls of the small intestine, and are absorbed into the bloodstream. The small intestine absorbs and disseminates most of the nutrients that are being released during the digestive process.

During the digestive process in the small intestine, the pancreas, the liver, and the gallbladder play essential roles, leading to the nutrients, now in their simplest chemical form, being able to be carried by the blood to all the cells of your body. These nutrients include amino acids for the creation of new cells, the rebuilding of organs, and restoring the muscle cells and fibers damaged by exercise. Some nutrients that are not immediately needed are stored by the liver, where they may be further processed and released when needed.

Pancreas, Liver, and Gallbladder

The pancreas produces digestive enzymes, which are reaction-starting catalytic proteins that break the carbohydrates, proteins, and fats of the foods in the small intestine into smaller molecules that can permeate the small intestine membranes and enter the bloodstream.

The liver performs numerous functions, including production and secretion of bile and cleansing the blood arriving from the small intestine. The bile that the liver produces passes through a passageway called the cystic duct into a small, pear-shaped organ, the gallbladder, where it is stored. When food arrives in the small intestine, contractions of the gallbladder deliver the bile to aid in the nutrient separations.

What is bile? This yellowish green-brown syrupy liquid is delivered from the gallbladder to the duodenum section of the small intestine to aid in the emulsification or breaking down of fats, leading to more effective digestion and absorption. The enzymes in bile break the fats into smaller pieces, and then into simpler, more digestible fatty acids. Bile also helps increase the contractions of peristalsis.

After its passage through the small intestine, remaining undigested foods and fluids, and older, expended cells from the GI tract, are delivered into the large intestine.

Large Intestine

Also called the colon, the large intestine is thicker and shorter than the small intestine, averaging five to six feet in length, and coiled in horizontal and vertical sections: the cecum is the first part, where food enters from the ileum, followed by the right, or ascending colon, then food travels through the across, or transverse colon, then into the descending or right colon, and finally the food is deposited into the "S" shaped sigmoid colon, which terminates in the rectum.

At this stage, the food waste left over from the preceding digestive processes is primarily in a liquid or paste state as it enters the colon, but becomes solid, or partially solid as water is removed, and the waste becomes stool and moves along through the colon with peristalsis. The stool is composed of food remnants and bacteria, which help break it down and dispatch any harmful bacteria that may be present. The stool is stored in the sigmoid colon and then emptied into the rectum to prepare for elimination.

Rectum and Anus

When the sigmoid colon senses the stool is ready for elimination, it empties its contents into the rectum, an eight-inch long straight tube that connects the sigmoid colon and the anus. Sensors in the rectum send precise signals to the brain that alert you that something is there and potentially ready to be eliminated. These messages can help you distinguish if it's gas, something solid, or if it's stool, and whether there is an urgency for elimination. The brain assesses if the rectal contents are ready for release, and if so, the rectum contracts and its sphincter muscles relax so the stool can move into the anus. If for any reason, the release needs to be delayed, the rectal sphincters tighten and reduce the sensation of urgency, or immediacy.

The anus is where the stool exits the body and is constructed of an internal anal sphincter muscle, which keeps the stool from exiting while you're asleep, and an external sphincter which you control and relax consciously when you are ready. These two muscles are joined in constructing the anus by the muscles that form the pelvic floor. As with the tissues of the rectum, sensitive nerve endings in the anus further confirm whether the stool contents are ready for elimination, and are solid or liquid, or are gaseous.

Nutrition: The Basics of What You Eat

Let's conclude this review of the process of digestion with a brief examination of what exactly it is that you are digesting. What are the main food groups that you consume and digest every day, and what are their functions in your body?

There are three main food sources of nutrition: protein, carbohydrates, and fats. On average, we are made of 16% protein, 16% fat, and 6% carbohydrates and minerals. The rest is water. These percentages can vary based on diet, lifestyle, and activity levels. A person who is overweight or obese will have a higher level of fat, while a weightlifter may have a higher ratio of protein, and a lower percentage of fat. What do these different food groups do, and how much do you need?

Proteins

Proteins are the building block of our bodies, constructing every cell, every organ and muscle. Cells regenerate and need proteins each day. Whenever you move or exercise, the protein in the muscles breaks down, depending on the intensity of the exertion, and needs to be replaced. When muscles are subject to hard exercise, and allowed to rest for a day or two, the rebuilding process tends to build up a bit more than was damaged, leading over time to increased muscle bulk.

For growth and rebuilding, our bodies need complete proteins, which are made of 20 amino acids. Our bodies can produce 11 of those 20 amino acids, but nine must come from our diet, also called essential amino acids. Food sources of complete protein (containing all 20 amino acids) include beef, chicken, and other meats, fish, eggs, and dairy products. In other words, animal sources. Plant-sourced foods, except for soy, quinoa, and buckwheat, are deficient in some of the essential amino acids. But a vegan, who eats no animal-derived product can meet the full amino acid requirement by mixing plant foods that complement each other, like the combination of beans and rice. A vegetarian can benefit in the same way, as well as with dairy and egg products. Vegans need to be attentive to the protein values of their diet, to ensure the full 20 amino acids requirement is met. One gram of protein contains four calories.

Carbohydrates

Most people are surprised to learn that carbohydrates are the largest component of most diets, given the press articles and diet advertising that advocate "low carb diets." In reality, carbohydrates are the fuel that powers our body; the source of energy that enables every organ and muscle to operate. The reasons this food group is subject to so much criticism trace to a common tendency to consume an excess of carbohydrates that leads to obesity, and for many of the carbohydrates people consume coming from poor sources of nutrition, especially refined sugar. When carbohydrates are sourced from complete grains and cereals, nuts and seeds, fruits and vegetables, they are accompanied by vitamins, minerals, fiber, antioxidants, and other valuable nutrients essential to many recommended diets. In addition to providing needed carbohydrates, these plant-based foods also contain some protein, and in the case of nuts and seeds, also contain healthy fats and oils. Like protein, one gram of carbohydrates contains four calories.

Fats and Oils

Nature designed fats to store energy that is not immediately needed. There is no question that fats should be part of our diet, but it's the sources of these fats, and the quantity we consume, that are important to understand. Fats from meat and full-fat dairy products are considered undesirable because they are saturated, which, in simple terms, means they are full of hydrogen, which causes the levels of LDL ("bad") cholesterol to rise and contributes to heart disease. Saturated fats tend to be solid at room temperature. Fats that are liquid at room temperature are called oils.

In contrast, oils from certain plant sources are highly desirable from a health standpoint. Extra virgin olive oil and avocado oil are classified as monounsaturated, which contributes to a reduction of LDL cholesterol and an increase in HDL ("good") cholesterol. Oils from sunflower, corn, safflower, and other polyunsaturated oils are also beneficial. Recommendations from the American Heart Association limit saturated fat to 5% to 6% of total daily calories or about 13 grams.

Be careful of the quantities of oil consumed since oils are a concentrated storage source of energy and contain nine calories in one gram.

Good Practices

In subsequent chapters, we'll go deeper into the foods that should and should not be part of your diet, or any healthy diet, but in overall good practice, your preference should be less processed, more natural foods, more vegetables, fruits, and whole grains and cereals, and avoidance or at least reduction of sugar and other highly refined carbohydrates. Fats should be from monounsaturated and polyunsaturated plant sources, and not from meat and dairy-sourced saturated fats.

When you come to the sections on the FODMAP diet, there will be a full review of how to test which food sources are best for you. For example, certain vegetables may be highly regarded as beneficial and high in key nutrients but may not be agreeing with your digestive system.

For a change of pace, we'll head into a discussion of the microbiome, which is the relatively new field of nutrition and health that centers around trillions of bacteria in our guts.

Chapter 2:

Microbiome - An Army of Microbes Keeping You Healthy

Let's begin by revisiting Giulia Enders' quote from the Introduction, which summarizes the realization that there is something going on in our bodies that is affecting our health and well-being, and controlling our bodily functions in ways that we are still trying to understand:

> *"Everyday we live, and every meal we eat, influences the great microbial organ inside us - for better or for worse."*

The Unknown Microbial Army

In 2012, when Dr. Enders first presented her idea that an army of bacteria and other microbes live in our gut and affect our digestion, health, and immune systems, she ignited popular support, but the medical community was more cautious, even though it's been known since the 1970's that we are carrying these microbial passengers. But in recent years, increasing support from gastroenterologists and immune system scientists grew as clinical research verified the presence, magnitude, and extensive influence of the microbiome.

Are Gut Microbes Helpful or Harmful?

There are estimated to be at least 1,000 species of bacteria in our guts. Most of the microbes in the GI tract have specific roles to play, like cleaning the gut, getting rid of harmful bacteria and viruses, and helping with digestion. Some microbiota create hormones and neurotransmitters that are essential to the functioning of the brain. Analysis of gut contents indicates that 95% of gut bacteria are beneficial or neutral. There are some microbes in our guts that may be pathogens, which means they can cause disease, but they are in the distinct minority and are often neutralized by beneficial bacteria and even helpful viruses. Should any of these pathogens escape the gastroesophageal tract and enter the bloodstream, they will usually be detected and destroyed by the immune system's innate response, with white cells called phagocytes engulfing the unwelcome germs.

But we all know bad microbes can occasionally survive and make trouble in the gut. Food poisoning, like salmonella, can overwhelm the defenses and create havoc within the microbiome. If you have ever had a stomach virus, you know what it can do. Fortunately, these events are rare, while the "good" 95% continue their beneficial work day and night, like breaking down sugars to make them digestible, among many other functions. Your microbiome is also programming and calibrating your immune system, keeping it alert to an invasion of harmful bacteria and viruses.

Where Does the Microbiome Come From?

Acquisition of internal bacteria begins at birth. It is generally accepted that while babies do not acquire bacteria for the microbiome while in utero, during birth the bacteria are picked up within the birth canal. This has led to theories, backed up by some studies, that babies born by caesarian section are not endowed with the mother's microbiome, and have less effective immune systems, leading to susceptibility to asthma and type 1 diabetes, among other disorders.

More microbial members are acquired during the first two years from a diversity of sources like breast milk, and exposure to the environment. Presumably, anything that is eaten and not sterilized is a potential source of bacteria that will stay in the GI tract. As we grow through childhood, the foods we eat are increasingly varied, and so are the bacteria we are ingesting. Viruses that live in the gut may be ingested, while viruses that are inhaled are subject to the attention of the immune system. Over time, the microbiome grows if the conditions are favorable until the requisite population is reached, and the size of the microbiome stabilizes.

What Affects the Microbiome?

The character and functionality of the microbiome can change, based on the natural selection, or "survival of the fittest" that favors stronger microbes, while on the negative side, the introduction of external factors like antibiotics or other medications can reduce the size and vitality of the microbiota, at least temporarily.

Our diet plays an influential role in building and maintaining a healthy microbial population since certain foods nourish and sustain the bacteria, and other foods can set them back. When we get to the FODMAP diet, we will explore the role certain foods may have in boosting, or weakening your microbiome. You can be sure that any stomach or intestinal disorder can wreak havoc with the bacteria. This can be short term, but in the case of chronic disorders like IBS, IBD, or Crohn's, the disturbances can have long-standing detrimental effects on the microbes.

How many microbes are there? As mentioned above, there are at least 1,000 different bacterial species discovered so far. There are claims of bacteria and other microbes in our guts vastly outnumbering our cells, until a 2016 study found it's almost even; there are 1.3 bacteria for each one of our cells. Still, that's quite a large number to host. Of course, bacteria are far smaller than our cells; the microbiome is estimated to weigh between three and five pounds in aggregate. This ratio does not include viruses, which are numerous but much smaller than bacteria.

Each of us has a different microbiome profile or composition, and it is this difference that may explain why certain foods agree with one person, but not with another. The differences can be caused by our genes, our diet, and even our lifestyle. Rob Knight, human microbiome expert and professor at the University of California San Diego, says that differences in the composition of people's microbiomes might explain why you can eat rice, while your friend has a bad reaction despite both of you eating other similar items, being the same age, and having a similar overall physical condition.

The Microbiome and the Gut-Brain Axis

It's estimated that there is a continuous flow of information between the brain and the gut, with 10% of information coming from the brain and 90% of the nerve fibers, primarily the vagus nerve, carrying messages from the gut. The microbes in the gut can measure hormone levels, for example, letting the brain know whether it's time for an adjustment. New studies are proposing that there may be a correlation between intestinal disorders like IBD, Crohn's, depression, and anxiety. Your mood and state of mind come from within.

Heribert Watzke, a food scientist, has identified a "hidden brain" in our gut and cites the unexpected effects it has on our sensations and feelings. Watzke informs us that there are at least one hundred million neurons within the gut-brain axis. To be clear, no thinking or human reasoning is going on in the gut, despite any "gut feelings" we may have. But the conditions in the gut are detected by the microbiome and forwarded to the brain as signals for interpretation and response.

Bacteria is certainly not unique to our guts. A wide diversity of microorganisms exist on our skin, inside our mouth, and are lining various orifices like our nostrils and nasal passages, the vagina, and throughout our bodies. Bacteria are the most numerous, by far, but we also are host to archaea, which are single-celled organisms that evolved separately from bacteria, plus viruses and fungi. Some bacteria attack viruses, and there are other viruses that infect and destroy bacteria. Combined, this plethora of microscopic creatures are the human microbiota, with the vast majority in the gut, counting trillions in number, and collectively called the microbiome.

This army of trillions of microbes directly controls and influences the digestive process, as well as being able to affect your cardiovascular and mental health. It can cause changes in your body weight and influences your immune system's functionality. The microbiome can initiate the autoimmune system, when the body's defenses overreact and cause inflammation, leading to rheumatoid arthritis, or diabetes. Along with a range of physical and psychological issues, any immune system malfunctions can cause cancer, or fail to destroy embryonic cancer or mutant cells as they are forming.

Does the Microbiome Control Obesity?

Obesity is caused primarily by consuming and digesting more calories than we expend. If we eat more than we use, the leftover calories are stored as fat, even if they arrive in your GI tract as carbohydrates. One of the main contributing factors to overeating is a malfunction of the hormone leptin, which manages energy by controlling appetite and tells the brain when you've eaten enough. If the microbiome misreads the situation and does not inform the brain that you're full, you will be tempted to keep eating. The microbiome can also improve the efficiency of digestion, and help your body obtain the nutrients it needs with less calorie-rich foods.

Further studies are needed to determine if the microbiome can be manipulated to tell the body to eat less and burn more calories by influencing the metabolic rate. The urgency for progress is underscored by one-third of Americans being overweight, and another one-third is obese:

- With the census of the medical community that being overweight or especially being obese is detrimental to health and makes you susceptible to diabetes and cardiovascular disease, and many other disorders, it is important to be aware of your body mass index or BMI.
- A BMI of up to 24.9 is normal, 25 to 29.9 is overweight, and 30 and above is obese. You can find a free BMI calculator online, so you can see your current status and use it as a baseline to measure progress in any weight reduction

program you undertake along with the FODMAP diet.

Digestion to Support the Immune System

According to Harvard's T.H. Chan School of Public Medicine, the microbiota in our guts can stimulate our immune systems by synthesizing vitamins like the B complex. Vitamin B12, for example, can be formed only by enzymes present in bacteria and is not available in plant or animal sources. Vitamin D is also produced in the gut. Importantly, the microbiota assembles molecules to assemble amino acids, which are the building blocks of protein.

Simple sugars and other less complex carbohydrates, like lactose in milk, are digested and absorbed easily as they enter the duodenum, the first part of the small intestine. More complex carbohydrates, such as fiber and starches, need more time and digestive action and generally descend through the small intestine into the large. During this descent, the bacteria are producing digestive enzymes, which are catalysts that assist in breaking down the more complex foods.

Fiber is a very complex, long-chain carbohydrate that is usually in two forms: soluble, which digests easily, and insoluble, which as the name implies, does not digest easily if at all. Instead, bacterial enzymes ferment this tough fiber to convert it to short-chain fatty acids.

Now in a digestible and usable form, these fatty acids have nutrient value and are involved in muscle function.

The fatty acids produced by the bacterial enzymes may also help prevent some chronic diseases such as certain types of cancer, ulcerative colitis, diarrhea caused by antibiotics, Crohn's disease, and other bowel disorders. Further immune system support is provided by the microbiota's detection of pathogens that may arrive when we eat or drink contaminated items.

If you are interested in getting to know your microbiota in greater detail, you can check out these prominent bacterial families in your gut, including Bacteroides, Firmicutes, Prevotella, and Ruminococcus; found especially in the small intestine. These bacteria that prefer a low oxygen environment are called anaerobic and tend to congregate in the large intestine including Bifidobacterium, Clostridium, Lactobacillus, and Peptostreptococcus. You may recognize these bacteria strains since some are listed among the live cultures in yogurt, which you add to your microbiome with each serving.

These and other anaerobic bacteria are credited with suppressing invasive, potentially harmful bacteria by competing with them for nutrients, and denying access to mucus membranes in the intestines. These attachment sites are where immune system activity is prevalent, including the construction of antimicrobial proteins.

Do You Need Probiotics?

In the follow up to the widening public awareness of the microbiome, interest has grown in the concept of probiotics, which are live, beneficial bacteria cultures that are ingested and are generally believed to supplement the existing microbiome population in your gut. There are essentially two forms of probiotics available to you:

1. Bacteria that occur naturally in foods that have fermented. In addition to yogurt, you can naturally and inexpensively add beneficial bacteria to your gut with other bacterially-fermented foods including cottage cheese, sauerkraut, pickles, pickled vegetables, kimchi, tempeh, kefir, kombucha, and natto (a Japanese fermented form of soy). Many kinds of cheese contain beneficial bacteria, especially aged cheeses. It is important not to cook the foods, which would kill the live bacteria cultures.
2. Probiotic dietary supplements that claim to contain millions of live bacteria in each capsule are available in virtually every pharmacy and store that sells dietary supplements. The strains of bacteria being provided are listed on the package and can be quite expensive.

The question is whether these probiotics are needed. Medical professionals have few doubts that the bacteria from natural food sources, like yogurt and sauerkraut, may have some benefit and safe if the person's microbiome is already healthy and does not need supplemental infusions of Bifidobacterium and Lactobacillus bacterial colonies.

Naturally-sourced probiotics from foods are believed to assist our absorption of calcium, control spikes in blood sugar, ferment foods so they pass more quickly through the gut to prevent constipation, and help protect the tissues that line the gut. New studies are looking into whether probiotics can help manage gut diseases like irritable bowel syndrome and how it can play a role in controlling obesity.

The need for probiotics in supplement form is less conclusive, with the view that for a healthy person with no microbiome issues, there seems to be little need for probiotic supplements. But in certain cases, they may be a good idea. According to Dr. Allan Walker, Professor of Nutrition at Harvard's T.H. Chan School of Public Health, and despite conflicting reports, "Probiotics can be most effective at both ends of the age spectrum because that's when your microbes aren't as robust as they normally are" (2020). He adds that probiotic supplements can positively influence the large bacterial population during times of deficiency and may help during stress caused by severe diarrhea or when restoring bacteria following an antibiotic regimen.

But Dr. Walker emphasizes that except for these extreme circumstances of stress-induced bacterial insufficiency, taking a probiotic supplement regimen is probably not going to have an effect on those whose gut health is normal. It is of relevance to note that probiotic supplements are expensive relative to obtaining a boost of beneficial bacteria from your diet. Probiotic capsules are now a rapidly growing, multi-billion dollar business in this country. These products are categorized as food supplements by the FDA, which means they are not regulated and their claims have not yet been verified.

What Are Prebiotics?

On the shelves next to *pro*biotics you will find a separate category of supplements called *pre*biotics. These do not contain live bacterial cultures to add to your microbiome, but rather are nutrients targeted to feed and nourish the microbiota that you already have. Their reason for being is based on the assumption that our microbiomes are subject to stress, toxins, antibiotics, and other drugs and medicines, plus other disturbances, and need a nutritional boost. Prebiotics are composed primarily of insoluble fiber, which are complex carbohydrates that pass through the stomach and most of the small intestine without being digested by the usual onslaught of digestive acids and enzymes, and end up in the lower intestinal tract, where they are available for the microbes to feed on.

Do you need to take prebiotic supplements? A balanced, healthy diet that contains a diversity of foods should contain an adequate amount of fiber, both soluble and insoluble, that serve to nourish the microbiome without the need to take prebiotic supplements, for example:

- Apples, pears, oranges, bananas, and most unprocessed fruits and berries
- Lettuce, kale, spinach, broccoli, celery, carrots, potatoes, and most vegetables

- Oats, wheat, rice, quinoa, and other whole grain, unrefined cereals, and grains
- Legumes (beans), walnuts, pecans, other nuts, and seeds like flax and chia

The opinion on prebiotic supplements expressed by *Harvard T.H. Chan School of Public Health* (2020), echoes this perspective, saying that while there are supplements that contain prebiotic fibers, many foods are natural, healthful sources of prebiotic fibers that will benefit your microbiome. Caution is offered to moderate a sudden increase in dietary fiber, which can cause production of gas, or flatulence.

However, in a situation where your diet is deficient in fiber, and you are unable to increase your fiber intake through diet, prebiotics may be an option. Fiber supplements can also be recommended to relieve constipation, for example, psyllium husk, and bran.

Diseases Affected by the Microbiome

You have already seen that the microbiome can affect obesity, and is also considered to be able to prevent or reduce symptoms of many diseases, both inside the gastrointestinal system, as well as in other parts of the body. The next chapter will go into these diseases and conditions in detail, but the following are a preview of what's next.

Serious intestinal disorders, including irritable bowel syndrome (IBS), inflammatory bowel disease (IBD), and Crohn's disease can be caused, and potentially treated by the microbiome. These diseases have the common symptoms of severe abdominal pain caused by excessive gas and bloating, a condition caused by gut dysbiosis, which is caused by harmful microbes. While medical treatment is generally needed to reduce the symptoms, certain probiotic bacteria, including bifidobacterium and lactobacillus bacterial colonies, found in yogurt and other probiotic-rich foods, are able to reduce the symptoms. They may also prevent disease-causing bacteria from attaching to intestinal walls, and help shrink ducts in intestinal walls that result in leaky gut.

Gastroesophageal reflux disease (GERD), heartburn, and acid reflux are related and are symptomatic of excess acid rising up out of the stomach, bypassing the sphincter that is supposed to keep it contained. Symptoms can range from mild discomfort to severe irritation and ulceration of the esophagus. There are OTC and Rx medicines to treat GERD and acid reflux by reducing or blocking acid flow. In addition, the microbiome may be able to prevent or reduce symptoms based on dietary adjustments.

Celiac disease is an intolerance to gluten, a complex protein that is found in wheat, rye, spelt, barley, and some other grains, and which certain people are unable to digest. Celiac disease is believed to be limited to a small part of the U.S. population, mostly with Eastern European backgrounds, and who account for perhaps only 2 to 3% of the population. Yet due to misinformation, gluten-free products have become a dominant factor in the marketplace.

Clostridium difficile is a gastric infection caused by a strain of dangerous bacteria. It is generally treated by medications that destroy not only c. difficile. but many beneficial bacteria in the microbiome. An effective treatment to rapidly rebuild the population of beneficial bacteria is to introduce donor stool into the large intestine, where it is able reach the prebiotic fibers and successfully repopulate.

Cancer can develop in different parts of the GI tract. Esophageal cancer can result from untreated GERD, leading to long term acidic burning and irritation of the sensitive esophageal tissues. Gastric cancer may be caused by excessively strong hydrochloric acid in the stomach, or by too frequent discharges of stomach acid when there is insufficient food in the stomach to absorb it. Colon, rectal, and anal cancers are mostly affected by genetics, but may be caused or exacerbated by imbalances in the ratio of microbiota that reach these lower sections of the GI tract.

Heart disease may be caused by certain activities within the microbiome, and may also be prevented by more beneficial microbes. Nutrients and amino acids found in some meats and animal-derived proteins can be converted by some microbiota to trimethylamine N-oxide (TMAO), a chemical associated with causing blockages in arteries that can lead to heart attacks and strokes. But conversely, a study among 1,500 patients, cited in *Healthline* (2017), showed that certain microbiota induced elevated levels of HDL ("good") cholesterol, while lowering artery-clogging LDL cholesterol, and triglycerides, which are fats circulating in the blood.

Diabetes is caused by excess blood sugar, and studies among infants have found that elevated blood sugars levels are preceded by changes in the ratio of healthy to unhealthy microbes in the gut. Subsequent research shows that a healthy microbiome can control blood sugar and stop the onset of type 1 diabetes.

Brain health is directly affected by the microbiome. Some neurotransmitters, like serotonin, which is an antidepressant, are made principally in the gut by several species of bacteria. The gut and the brain are connected by the vagus nerve, which descends from the brainstem and influences a wide range of functions, plus millions of other neurons that alert the brain to the state of the gut, and prompt the brain to take remedial action when required. The microbial profile of people with psychological disorders is different from the profile of healthy persons, and may have an influence on mental health. Other research shows a relationship between the composition of the microbiome and depression, leading to further studies that would treat depression with probiotics.

Future Microbiome Research

The microbiome is not a static, unchanging entity; rather it is a living, dynamic collective organism that changes on a daily or longer basis, being affected by diet, health, stress, medication, and even exercise. It's role in influencing our health is already well appreciated, yet is far from fully understood, and science is still in early stages of grasping the full extent of the microbiome in affecting many different aspects of our physical health and mental condition.

We need to understand much more about the complex range of interactions between the microbiome and its human host, which is challenging, since the bacteria and viruses cannot be observed directly. The subjects of greatest interest include:

- The degree of influence exerted on health, and on the formation of diseases by the metabolic substances (metabolites) that are produced by the microbiome, and to determine if the microbiome can be manipulated to resist disease, more effectively neutralize pathogens, and improve the body's response to medications.
- How the microbiome environment achieves a state of balance, or equilibrium, and what factors can cause it to become unbalanced.
- The potential for probiotic foods and supplements to significantly enhance the viability and role of the microbiome, and the regulatory implications of prescribing customized probiotic bacterial colonies.
- How the state and composition of the microbiome varies between healthy people and those with various types of chronic diseases, including gastrointestinal disorders, and also extending to diabetes, cardiovascular disease, obesity, and cancer.

- How the microbiome of women during pregnancy is affected, especially if the composition of the microbial community changes during this period, and also to learn how the microbiome evolves in infants and children.
- Whether diseases can be identified in their earliest stages of development by discovering how to detect diagnostic biomarkers in the microbiome.
- If the composition and functionality of the microbiome can be changed and improved through transplantation of gut bacteria from donors.
- How the microbiome may affect mood and state of mind, through impulses carried by the vagus nerve, a two-way neural highway that runs from our brain to various organs in the body, including the gut.

Now we can learn what your gut may be telling you. We'll look into the various digestive diseases and disorders in greater detail.

Chapter 3:

What Is Your Gut Telling You?

Your gut is unique in many ways from other parts of your body. You are aware of your GI tract whenever you are hungry, and sense the enjoyment of eating and tasting foods. You know when you may have eaten a bit too much, and may feel indigestion, cramps, gas and bloating. If you suffer from any of the more serious gastroesophageal or gastrointestinal diseases, you are even more conscious, due to the disruptions and discomforts they can cause on a daily basis.

You are also able to have a direct effect on your digestive system by varying what you eat. In an extreme example, an overly spicy food can gain your immediate attention in its passage from mouth to throat to esophagus to stomach. An antacid like calcium carbonate can bring almost immediate relief to heartburn and indigestion. Changes in your diet can have considerable effect in causing, or in relieving, many symptoms of digestive disorders, which is what the FODMAP chapters of this book will be discussing.

Signs of potential gastroesophageal and gastrointestinal problems:

- Bleeding during bowel movements
- Bloating and gas
- Constipation
- Diarrhea
- Heartburn and indigestion
- Incontinence
- Nausea and vomiting
- Pain in the abdomen
- Swallowing difficulty
- Unexplained weight gain or loss

Chronic Disorders and You

If left untreated, these relatively mild conditions can develop into chronic disorders, or may be signals that something is amiss and needs attention. In this section, we will explain these disorders in depth, so you can recognize and understand the symptoms and causes, and become familiar with how these disorders are currently being treated.

Important disclaimer: The information in this section, and throughout this book, is for educational purposes only, and is not intended to offer medical advice, or to diagnose, treat, cure, or prevent any disease, condition, or illness.

Acid Reflux, Heartburn, and GERD

We begin with one of the most frequent gastrointestinal and gastroesophageal disorders. GERD is the blanket term that describes a chronic form of acid reflux, which is when digestive acid from the stomach backs up into the esophagus. Normally, the gastroesophageal sphincter, which is at the base of the esophagus, opens only to allow food to enter the stomach, and then closes tightly to prevent food and acid from leaking back up into the esophagus. Unlike the stomach walls, which are reinforced to withstand the strong acid, the walls of the esophagus are easily irritated, burned, scarred and damaged by repeated exposure to the acids.

Since 60% of American adults experience indigestion and occasional acid reflux, it is likely that you may be among this majority. It can occur at any time, even on an empty stomach; any time the stomach excretes acid, and some of it leaks upward into the esophagus. If the acid is strong enough, it may irritate the walls of the stomach, and cause distress without having to reach the esophagus. For example, one possible cause of this effect can be chewing gum on an empty stomach, which causes acid to be generated, but without food in the stomach to absorb it.

Heartburn is the term many people use to describe the painful sensation of acid reflux, and has no relationship to the heart. GERD is the diagnosis for when mild acid reflux occurs once a week or more, or when it is moderate or severe, and occurs twice weekly, or more often. GERD is a chronic condition, meaning it is continuing, over time.

Symptoms of GERD may include a range of discomforts, some of which may be painful, including chest pain, often described as a burning sensation, or heartburn. It may be suspected as a heart attack, and if it does not respond to antacids, a call to the doctor or visit to the Emergency Room may be necessary.

On occasion, stomach acid and sour, partially digested food may be regurgitated, coming back through the esophagus to the mouth and throat, and requiring a thorough rinse with water. Other symptoms of GERD may be difficulty swallowing or a sensation of a lump caught in the throat. Many GERD symptoms are experienced at night, and may be accompanied by a cough or laryngitis. Nighttime GERD events can be very disruptive to sleep. Asthma symptoms may occur.

There are three levels of over-the-counter (OTC) medications to treat GERD:

Antacids, like Tums®, and Rolaids® are for immediate relief of symptoms. They contain calcium carbonate, which works within a minute or two to neutralize the acidity and stop, or appreciably reduce, the most severe discomfort. These treatments are short term and may need to be repeated. Antacids do not offer preventative effects, unless taken with the food, and even then, are short term in effect.

H2 receptor blockers provide preventative effects; one tablet taken in the morning protects throughout the day, and one in the evening provides nighttime protection. Package instructions recommend taking the tablet 30 minutes before eating foods that might lead to acid reflux and heartburn. Our bodies produce histamine to stimulate acid production in the stomach. H2 blockers work by occupying receptor cells and preventing acid-producing parietal cells from responding to the histamine, which reduces acid secretion in your stomach.

The popular brands of H2 blockers function similarly, and include famotidine, sold as Pepcid® and Pepcid AC® (which includes an antacid for immediate effects), cimetidine, sold as Tagamet®, and ranitidine, sold as Zantac®, although Zantac is currently off the market due to FDA concerns over one of its ingredients. These medications were originally Rx, requiring a prescription, but are now widely available as OTC. Pharmacy chains also offer less expensive generic versions, since the brand patents have expired.

Proton Pump Inhibitors (PPIs) are considered to be the most potent inhibitors of stomach acid secretions, making them the most effective preventative of the symptoms of GERD. PPIs were introduced as prescription medications, but are now available as OTC; popular brands include lansoprazole, sold as Prevacid®, omeprazole, sold as Prilosec®, and esomeprazole, known as Nexium®. They are recommended in cases of hard-to-control GERD symptoms, and both to prevent and treat ulcers in the stomach and the duodenum (where most ulcers develop).

PPIs block production of hydrogen ions, a positively charged hydrogen atomic nucleus (a proton is the nucleus of a hydrogen atom, and combines with chlorine and other chemicals to form hydrochloric acid, which is the digestive acid in our stomachs).

PPIs have come under scrutiny for possible interactions with other drugs, including the blood thinner clopidogrel, known as Plavix®, and users of PPIs are advised to check with doctors or pharmacists about other medications they are taking. A more recent concern involves possible kidney damage from prolonged usage of PPIs, and the drug is now directed to be used for a single treatment phase of one tablet per day for 14 days, followed by a four month hiatus, and then followed by two more similar cycles. To conform with this FDA directive, branded and generic versions of the OTC PPIs are packaged in a box containing three bottles of 14 tablets, with clear instructions to not exceed 14-day usage, and the need to wait four months before another cycle.

Lifestyle changes can help relieve the onset of acid reflux: eating smaller meals, not eating a large meal before going to bed, identifying and avoiding foods that may not agree with you, which can include spicy and fried foods, alcohol, chocolate, coffee and tea. Each of us may have sensitivities to other foods that can cause an acid reflux attack. The FODMAP diet may play a pivotal role in rooting out foods that trigger indigestion caused by acid reflux, enabling to eliminate or reduce only foods specific to your sensitivities, instead of a blanket elimination of every possible culprit! Raising the head end of your bed by six to 10 inches may help reduce the risk of nighttime acid reflux; alternatively, use two pillows, angled to raise your upper body.

Speak to your doctor if your GERD symptoms do not respond well to the OTC medications, or if you find yourself needing antacids in addition to H2 blockers or

PPIs. Your condition may require stronger prescription medications, or other treatments. It may be necessary to be checked physically for existing gastroesophageal or gastrointestinal ulcers. The customary procedure to check for ulcers, inflammation, scarring and other damage is an endoscopy examination of your GI tract:

- The gastroenterologist lower a long tube into your mouth, down your throat and into your esophagus.
- A very small video camera attached to the end of the tube lets the doctor examine your esophagus, the esophageal sphincter, your stomach, and your small intestine.
- Anything that is seen that looks suspicious can be biopsied, by removing a small sample of tissue to analyze for damage.

You'll be sedated during the endoscopy procedure, which does not take long, and is performed on an outpatient basis, meaning you'll go home soon after you wake up. Many gastroenterologists like to conduct a colonoscopy at the same time, for the convenience of you being sedated and in an operating room.

Celiac Disease

As you will have read in the previous chapter, celiac disease is a potentially serious disorder, primarily caused by gluten in baked goods and cereals, and that can bring gastrointestinal discomfort to people. While celiac disease can cause intestinal damage and other complications, and should be taken seriously, it is surprisingly of concern to a disproportionate share of the population: results of a recent survey published by CBS News (2020) shows that it affects 1.8 million American adults, or less than 2% of the adult U.S. population. The disorder affects a range of genetic and ethnic profiles, but has a particular concentration among people of Eastern European, Ashkenazi Jewish descent. The survey also revealed that the percentage of Americans afflicted with celiac disease has increased fourfold in the past 50 years, although this may be a function of greater awareness, leading to more diagnoses.

According to the Mayo Clinic, celiac disease or gluten-sensitive enteropathy, is an immune reaction to consumption of gluten, a complex protein most often found in cereals like wheat, spelt, barley and rye. In addition to occurring naturally in these grains, some bakers add more gluten to bread dough to give the bread structure. Gluten is activated and intensified by kneading, which further raises the gluten content.

Gluten in the diet initiates an immune response in the small intestine of persons with celiac disease. Short term or immediate symptoms can include stomach ache, gas and bloating, and diarrhea, and over time, the body's reaction can become serious, with damage to the lining of the small intestine. This can cause malabsorption, which is inability of the small intestine to absorb certain nutrients. Results of malabsorption can include fatigue, loss of weight, diarrhea, anemia, and bloating. In time, these complications can become serious. In addition to these symptoms, celiac disease-induced malabsorption in children can limit growth and physical development.

There is no known cure for celiac disease, but the symptoms can be reduced or eliminated in most cases by following a strict gluten-free diet. This is becoming easier now given the proliferation of gluten-free products that have entered the market. On a related note, the same CBS News report indicates that nearly 2 million Americans are following a gluten-free diet, despite not being diagnosed with celiac disease.

How do you get this disease? Celiac disease is most often inherited, as your genes make you sensitive to certain foods, notably wheat and other cereals containing gluten. Other factors may cause celiac disease, only some of which have been identified:

- Infections in the gut, and certain strains of bacteria among the colonies within the microbiota may have an effect.
- A woman may develop celiac sensitivities during pregnancy or childbirth, or during the time she is feeding an infant.
- It may be the result of a viral infection, or even as a consequence of your body's reaction to extreme stress. Your body may overreact to gluten in bread, or pasta or a bagel you eat, or any food containing wheat or rye, for example.

- Susceptibility to developing celiac disease may also be among those who have type 1 diabetes, Down's or Turner's syndrome, Addison's disease, microscopic or lymphocytic colitis, or have a close relative with celiac disease or dermatitis herpetiformis.

Celiac disease can be more than uncomfortable and may have serious physical implications. Your small intestine is lined with tiny hairlike projections called villi, which are essential to absorption of food-derived nutrients, vitamins, and minerals. Celiac disease can cause these villi to shrink, which retards or prevents absorption of these key nutrients, leading to a range of symptoms like malnutrition:

- Malnutrition is one of the most common consequences of celiac disease, and occurs when the disease goes untreated, or fails to respond to a gluten-free diet.
- Malnutrition can lead to weight loss, and anemia, and in children, it can cause slow growth and development.
- Bone weakening and a tendency to breakage can result from osteoporosis developing in adults as a consequence of failure to absorb sufficient amounts of calcium and vitamin D.
- Inability to absorb calcium and vitamin D may also lead to reproductive issues, including infertility and miscarriages.

- Lactose intolerance may also be caused by celiac disease; it is the inability to digest lactose, the natural sugar in milk and other dairy products, and results in severe abdominal pain, and diarrhea. A person who practices the FODMAP diet will be instructed to switch to lactose-free dairy products during the initial phase.
- Nervous system malfunctions can be caused, including seizures, and peripheral neuropathy, which affects the nerves of the hands and feet.
- Refractory and nonresponsive celiac disease is when the symptoms continue, despite switching to a gluten-free diet. This may be the result of some gluten still remaining, unknown, in the diet, or might be caused by colitis, irritable bowel syndrome, pancreatic malfunction, or residual pathogenic bacteria in the small intestine.

Speak to your doctor if the symptoms of celiac disease do not respond to a strict gluten-free diet after six months, or at any time you find the symptoms to be uncomfortable and interfering with your lifestyle. Your gastroenterologist may order a blood test for antibodies or to create a genetic profile to diagnose if you have celiac disease, since many people with celiac disease don't know they have it. Two blood tests can help diagnose whether you have celiac disease:

- Serology testing examines your blood for antibodies, and looks for antibody proteins that signal that gluten is triggering an immune response.

- Genetic testing checks for HLA-DQ2 and HLA-DQ8, which are human leukocyte antigens that can indicate if celiac disease is present.

Be careful to avoid interfering with the test results: have the blood test before going on a gluten-free diet; otherwise the absence of gluten reaction could cause a false negative finding.

As a follow up to the blood test, or very possibly as a first step, the gastroenterologist may order an endoscopy test, which is a visual examination of your GI tract. As was explained above regarding GERD, the doctor extends a long tube down your throat and into your esophagus. A tiny video camera at the end of the tube allows the specialist to visually examine your esophagus, the esophageal sphincter, the stomach, and your small intestine. Anything suspicious can be biopsied, by removing a small sample of tissue to analyze for damage to the villi or any other parts of the GI tract. You'll be sedated during this process, which does not take long, and is performed on an out-patient basis, meaning you'll go home soon after you wake up.

A new technology, called a capsule endoscopy, involves swallowing a pill-sized camera that transmits images as it passes through the digestive system. This does not require sedation, but it is of limited application at this time.

Chronic Constipation

Most of us experience constipation at some time in our lives; we describe it as infrequent bowel movements, or hard stools that are difficult to pass, and cause us to strain. Some think that constipation is incomplete emptying during a bowel movement. From the gastroenterologist's perspective, fewer than three bowel movements per week, or hard, difficult-to-pass stools at least 25% of the time are the most common confirmations of constipation.

In all cases, constipation involves not having regular, comfortable bowel movements, and is among the most common chronic gastrointestinal disorders that doctors treat, with over 2.5 million Americans seeking medical assistance annually for constipation, and spending close to 800 million dollars on laxatives, stool softeners, and other treatments.

But what is chronic constipation and what makes it different from acute constipation?

- Acute constipation is short term, lasting for a few days, and usually due to travel disruptions in routine, medication, change of diet, illness, stopping an exercise routine, or a reduction of fiber in the diet. Acute constipation generally responds well to short term use of OTC laxatives, resumption of exercise, or increasing dietary fiber.
- Chronic constipation is longer lasting, continuing for weeks, months, or even longer,

with only partial results from OTC laxatives, and the need to take them continuously; prescription medications may be needed. Adding fiber to the diet is of minimal effect. Chronic constipation is disruptive to normal activities, with days of discomfort followed by urgency to find a toilet when the laxative effect finally kicks in.

People most susceptible to chronic constipation tend to be female, over age 65, and do not exercise regularly, or may be confined to bed for a prolonged period. People with Parkinson's disease may experience constipation because the disorder can interfere with peristalsis, and its action of moving food through the digestive system. Pregnant women can be subject to bouts of long lasting constipation. With all of that said, frankly, it can happen to anyone.

Causes of chronic constipation vary and include:

- Dysfunction of the muscles that form the pelvic floor, and normally would be involved with rectal muscle contractions.
- Diabetes, hypothyroidism, and other endocrine or metabolic disorders. Multiple sclerosis, Parkinson's (see above re: peristalsis), and other neurological disorders, as well as spinal cord damage, and among those who have suffered a stroke.
- Irregularities in the colon, including bowel strictures, and tears in the rectum and anus.

- Constipation may be caused by depression, and other mental issues, including eating disorders, chronic anxiety, and long term stress.
- Bowel diseases, including Crohn's, irritable bowel disease, and inflammatory bowel syndrome (discussed below), and diverticulitis.

Constipation may also be in response to a wide range of medications, including opiate-based painkillers, diuretics, anticholinergics, calcium channel blockers and other medications that contain calcium, including OTC antacids, plus anti-diarrhea treatments, antipsychotics, antidepressants, and antihistamines.

Diet is often the go-to suspected cause, and the first recommendation, before medications, and other lifestyle adjustments, is to drink more water, and eat more fiber. When we get to the FODMAP diet, there will be an explanation how constipation may be treated by eliminating certain foods from your diet, or adding others. But it is not always possible to know the causes of chronic constipation, a situation described as chronic idiopathic constipation.

Self-treatment usually begins with OTC laxatives based on a natural extract from the senna root which stimulates a bowel movement within 24 to 48 hours. Hard stools can be treated with stool softeners, which use polyethylene glycol, an osmotic that causes bowels to absorb water, to soften and pass more easily. A completely natural fiber-based treatment is based on psyllium husk, and is best known as Metamucil®. There are store-brand generic versions of these OTC brands.

Visit your doctor for a gastrointestinal diagnosis if you are becoming dependent on laxatives and stool softeners, and need to take them continuously. The doctor may ask you about your bowel movements, and you will need to describe your bowel habits in detail. The doctor will probably use diagnostic tests to learn what's causing the constipation. You may be instructed to stop taking some constipation-inducing medications. Rx medications may be prescribed, including those approved by the FDA such as lubiprostone (Amitiza®), and linaclotide (Linzess®), and have been demonstrated in clinical trials to effectively and safely alleviate the symptoms of chronic constipation.

On a more urgent basis, see your doctor immediately if you see blood in your stool, or experience unexplained weight loss, or suffer from extreme pain with your bowel movements.

Crohn's Disease

Crohn's disease is defined as an inflammatory bowel disorder that is not limited to one digestive tract zone, but may affect any part of the gastrointestinal tract, extending from the mouth to the rectum and anus, although some people's symptoms are limited to the colon.

Those who suffer from Crohn's may complain of a wide range of signs and symptoms, including abdominal pain and distension, weight loss, fever, and diarrhea. Some complications can extend beyond the GI tract, including anemia, arthritis, skin rashes, fatigue, and inflammation of the eye. It may cause loss of appetite and weight loss, and limited digestion of nutrients, all of which can lead to malnutrition. Symptoms of Crohn's may come on suddenly, then disappear for a time. Variations in diet can trigger symptoms. In this context, Crohn's is one of several different types of inflammatory bowel disease (IBD).

Earlier belief that Crohn's is caused by dietary factors and stress has given way to new findings: diet and stress may aggravate Crohn's symptoms, but the causes are now believed to be hereditary, and immune system disorders:

- People who have family members with Crohn's are more likely to acquire the disease, strongly suggesting it is genetically passed among relatives, but in the majority of cases, genetics do not play a role, so heredity is a secondary factor.
- Doctors suspect that rogue bacteria or viruses in the gut trigger autoimmune responses, causing the immune system to attack intestinal lining cells, and other cells within the digestive transact. However, the suspected malevolent bacteria and viruses have not yet been identified, and cannot be isolated for destruction through medicine.

According to the Mayo Clinic (2020), there are several risk factors for Crohn's that you should know about:

- While Crohn's can begin at any age, it tends to begin when people are below 30.
- Ethnicity does not limit who can develop Crohn's.
- As noted above, if you have family members with Crohn's, you have a greater possibility of developing symptoms.
- Smoking is considered to be a prime factor for causing Crohn's, and for intensifying the symptoms.
- Be careful with NSAIDs (non-steroidal anti-inflammatory drugs), which are popular pain relievers like ibuprofen, naproxen (Aleve®) and aspirin, which are anti-inflammatory in small doses, but frequent use can aggravate the esophagus, stomach, and intestines, exacerbating the symptoms of Crohn's.

In addition to the discomforts and lifestyle disruptions that Crohn's can cause, untreated, it can lead to serious complications, including:

- Bowel obstruction from scarring and narrowing of the intestinal wall.
- Ulcers, which are open sores caused by chronic inflammation, and that can occur throughout the entire digestive tract. Ulcers can advance to become fistulas, which are complete openings, allowing fluids to travel from the intestines to other parts of the body, even causing anal

fissures. Fistulas can become infected and potentially life-threatening.
- Malnutrition and weight-loss can become a result of abdominal pain, cramping and diarrhea, making it hard to eat normal quantities and limiting the intestines' ability to absorb key nutrients. Low absorption of iron and vitamin B_{12} can lead to anemia.
- Colon cancer risk is increased by Crohn's disease. While regular colon screenings (colonoscopy) are recommended generally after age 50, those with Crohn's should check with their doctors if the screening should take place earlier, and more frequent. Polyps of concern that are detected during the screening can be removed at that time to be biopsied. As mentioned, gastroenterologists often recommend conducting the colonoscopy and the gastroesophageal endoscopy examination of the upper GI tract.
- Blood clots are believed to occur more often among those with Crohn's, and if your doctor thinks you may be at risk, a blood thinner may be prescribed.

There is no cure for Crohn's disease currently, but treatments and therapies are able to promote healing of tissues damaged by inflammation, manage symptoms and put the disease into remission, at least for a time.

Drugs and medications for Crohn's tend to be tailored to individual needs, or personalized, so each person's treatment may be unique. Crohn's disease often goes in cycles of flare-ups followed by remission, so treatment plans will vary at certain times, and require monitoring. The goal of these medications is to lower the body's immune response, reduce inflammation, and calm the body's defenses so the digestive system can recover from the onslaught:

- **Corticosteroids** are steroids that are used on a short term basis to lower inflammation and lower the immune response. Common corticosteroids are budesonide, hydrocortisone, methylprednisolone, and prednisone. These drugs are prescribed with caution, given the side effects which can include glaucoma, high blood pressure, weight gain, and mood swings. Liver damage or osteoporosis can occur if taken for more than three months.
- **Aminosalicylates** are also prescribed for ulcerative colitis, these drugs are believed to lower inflammation of the lining of the intestine, and reduce or eliminate symptoms. Side effects can be headaches, nausea and vomiting, diarrhea, and heartburn. The kidneys may need to be monitored to avoid damage, and blood tests are used to ensure the white blood count remains stable and doesn't fall too low.

- **Immunomodulators** are medications that may be prescribed if corticosteroids and aminosalicylates are not effective, or if fistulas develop. These medications can help keep a patient with Crohn's or ulcerative colitis stay in remission, and may also help heal fistulas. Examples of these medications are azathioprine (Imuran®), mercaptopurine (Purinethol®), cyclosporine (Gengraf®, Neoral®, Sandimmune®), and methotrexate. Possible side effects are the same as for the aminosalicylates.
- **Biologics** are drugs for people with moderate to severe Crohn's, and work to lower inflammation in the lining of the intestines. They do not suppress the entire immune system; just specific areas. Biologics may be prescribed if symptoms are moderate or severe, or if other treatments are ineffective. They can help a patient taper off their use of steroids. The most commonly used biologics are anti-tumor necrosis factor-alpha therapies, anti-integrin therapies, anti-interleukin-12, and interleukin-23 therapy. Side effects are similar to the preceding medications, plus low blood pressure, and a low risk of toxic reaction, or susceptibility to infections.
- Other medications can include antibiotics to control excessive bacterial growth in the gut, and loperamide, an antidiarrheal drug taken short term to control severe diarrhea.

Many people can be helped to function normally with Crohn's disease through lifestyle and dietary modifications:

Since the GI tract contains a vast population of bacteria, some people take probiotics to introduce new bacteria to improve the balance, which may be out of kilter. As has been described above, probiotics may be ingested in sauerkraut, yogurt, kefir, cheeses, and other foods containing live bacteria cultures, or probiotics may be taken as dietary supplement capsules. But do probiotics work? Researchers have analyzed several species of probiotic bacteria that hold potential, including bifidobacterium, which is in yogurt among other sources, but more studies are underway to confirm effectiveness.

Fish oil is considered a possible aid in relieving inflammation due to high content of omega-3 fatty acids. Research is not conclusive, but fish oil capsules are safe to try.

Taking digestive pressures off the stomach and intestines by switching to a liquid diet for a week, or several weeks, can let these organs rest, and may prevent symptoms while the GI tract resets itself. During the liquid diet, gastric inflammation may be able to subside. It's important that the liquid diet be complete in providing necessary carbohydrates, proteins, fats, minerals, vitamins, and other essential nutrients. To play it safe, this type of treatment should be undertaken under medical supervision.

Since stress can be a trigger of Crohn's symptoms, practicing yoga may help. Yoga emphasizes posture and breathing, and is a time-tested way to relax. Yoga may be practiced at home, or in a group setting with the guidance and support of a trained yoga instructor. Studies have confirmed that yoga may be an effective, safe part of your treatment, and in fact, any exercise that relieves stress can similarly be of value in helping calm the intestines.

Turmeric is a popular spice that contains curcumin, which is believed to reduce inflammation, although research has been limited to small-scale studies. Some users are convinced that turmeric helps relieve symptoms of Crohn's, as well as of ulcerative colitis, but additional research is needed. It's safe to use, but in excess could cause digestive irritation. It's available in tablets and capsules, and as a tea and extract.

Camel's milk may come as a surprise, and hard to find, but if you are not meeting your nutritional needs due to Crohn's, this may be of value. It's rich in calcium, iron, magnesium, zinc, and copper, plus vitamins A, B2, C, and E, while being low in cholesterol and fat. Camel's milk contains antioxidants and proteins that can reduce inflammation, so it may help relieve Crohn's symptoms. However, additional studies are required for verification.

Biofeedback is a technique that helps you to control physical responses with conscious thoughts, and is recognized as effective in reducing stress and anxiety. Electrical sensors provide feedback on your heart and breathing rates, brain waves, and other bodily functions. With training you can learn to manage those functions, by relaxing certain muscles or modifying your breathing, bringing stress under your control, and helping manage Crohn's symptoms.

Medical cannabis is being studied to determine if it can calm the symptoms of Crohn's and other bowel disorders, but no verifiable findings have been published.

It's time to see a doctor when you are experiencing prolonged, intense abdominal pain, continuous nausea and vomiting, ongoing diarrhea that does not stop when taking OTC medications, or when you see blood in your stool. Also see your doctor if your stomach or intestinal discomfort is accompanied by a fever that lasts for more than one or two days.

Inflammatory Bowel Disease and Irritable Bowel Syndrome

Is there a difference between inflammatory bowel disease (IBD) and irritable bowel syndrome (IBS)? And are they distinctive from Crohn's disease, and ulcerative colitis? It seems like these diseases have many of the same symptoms, and may be treated in some of the same ways. All of these diseases can cause abdominal discomfort and pain, and diarrhea, and may lead to malnutrition and weight loss if not treated. As you will see, Crohn's disease and ulcerative colitis fall under the same grouping. Although symptoms of inflammatory bowel disease and irritable bowel syndrome appear similar, they have different causes, and they vary in intensity and frequency. Let's take a closer look.

Inflammatory Bowel Disease

As the name implies, IBD includes disorders and immune responses that cause inflammation of the gastrointestinal tract. Inflammatory bowel disease is the blanket term for a group of inflammatory conditions which affect and inflame the digestive tract, principally Crohn's disease and ulcerative colitis:

- Crohn's disease, which we've covered in depth in the previous section, may affect any segment or place within the gastrointestinal tract. But, this version of IBD most frequently impacts the small intestine and the first section of the large intestine, or colon. Crohn's disease may cause areas of inflammation that can impart damage to several layers of the intestinal tract wall.
- Ulcerative colitis occurs further down the digestive tract, by causing inflammation of the large intestine, or colon, and the rectum. But while Crohn's disease can do damage to multiple layers of the small intestinal wall, the effects of ulcerative colitis are limited to damaging the innermost layer of the large intestinal wall.

Crohn's disease is generally more severe in its symptoms than ulcerative colitis, but occurs far less frequently. As reported in *Pharmacy & Therapeutics*

(2014), there were 1.86 billion cases of ulcerative colitis worldwide, but just 1.3 million verified cases of Crohn's disease.

Inflammatory bowel disease—both Crohn's disease and ulcerative colitis—is currently without a cure. It is a long-term condition, whose symptoms are responsive to various types of treatments.

Symptoms of IBD include diarrhea, bloody stools, rectal bleeding, sudden bowel movement urges, cramps and abdominal pain, as well as weight loss.

Diagnosis of IBD may be performed by X-ray or CT to enable the doctor to see inside the GI tracts and look for signs of damage. Alternatively, endoscopy and colonoscopy examinations may be conducted (explained previously). Blood tests can reveal signals of inflammation, and stool examinations can also reveal problems.

Treatment of IBD is designed to put symptoms into remissions, and a range of medications are available, as presented in the section on Crohn's disease, and include immunomodulators, aminosalicylates, and biologics.

Irritable Bowel Syndrome

IBS is also a long-term disease that affects the small and large intestines, and results in a range of digestive disorders. But unlike IBD, IBS does not result in visible damage or signs of inflammation in the digestive tract. IBS is more common than Crohn's disease within IBD, affecting about 12% of adults. It occurs more frequently among women, and among those below the age of 50. As with IBD, the causes of IBS are unknown, but are suspected to be caused by other digestive issues, and may be brought on by prolonged stress, or depression. There may be genetic causes, as well.

Symptoms of IBS include the usual abdominal cramps and pain, bloating caused by excess gas, feeling of incomplete bowel evacuation, and mucus in the stool.

Diagnosis of IBS will usually begin with a discussion with the doctor about symptoms, and about the frequency and types of bowel movements. No tests currently exist to precisely identify IBS, but blood tests, stool tests, endoscopy or colonoscopy may be ordered to rule out other conditions. A test for lactose intolerance involves a hydrogen breath test.

Treatment of IBS may include medications, such as the anti-diarrheal drug loperamide (Imodium®), laxatives like ExLax® and Senokot®, antispasmodics, fiber supplements like Metamucil®, and antidepressants, which may be prescribed to reduce abdominal pain and cramps. Lifestyle modification may be recommended, including a high fiber diet, avoidance of gluten, exercising regularly, managing stress through yoga and meditation, and ensuring good sleep habits

Food Intolerance

Food intolerances are common, and on the rise worldwide, with an estimated 20% of the global population affected. Unlike some of the gastrointestinal diseases we've been discussing, food intolerances tend to be less serious, but still can cause a wide range of unpleasant or disturbing symptoms. Frequently, food intolerances are hard to diagnose, which is why the FODMAP diet is a valuable way to weed out intolerances by process of elimination. Elimination diets remove foods that conceivably are causes of intolerances for a period until symptoms disappear or significantly diminish. Then the questionable foods are reintroduced individually while keeping alert for the return of symptoms

Food intolerances are one type of food hypersensitivity; food allergies are another, different type of hypersensitivity. The symptoms of both may be similar, requiring a doctor's tests to determine which type of hypersensitivity you are experiencing. Food allergies cause immune system responses; food intolerances do not.

Symptoms of food intolerance include some associated with IBD and IBS such as diarrhea, bloating and gas, abdominal pain, constipation, and acid reflux or GERD. Other symptoms may include nausea and vomiting, fatigue, headaches, runny or stuffy nose, and skin disorders, like rashes, hives, and flushing.

Common intolerances include these most common causes:

- **Dairy** can cause digestive disorders, usually due to intolerance to lactose, which is a form of sugar; the shortage of lactase enzymes makes lactose difficult to digest. Lactose-free milk and other dairy products are widely available, and dairy products that are fermented, like kefir and yogurt, tend to be more digestible.
- **Gluten** can cause intolerance due to celiac disease, which is discussed in detail in a previous section. Gluten is a protein found in wheat, rye, spelt, and other grains. Some bread and other baked products have additional gluten added. While celiac disease is limited to less than 2% of the U.S. population, a larger segment of the population, up to 13% may experience non celiac gluten sensitivity. gluten-free bread and baked products are increasing in popularity, even among those not sensitive to gluten.
- **Caffeine,** which is found in coffee, tea, chocolate, soft drinks, and energy drinks, is appreciated for its stimulant effect. This unique quality is due to its blocking of receptors for adenosine, a neurotransmitter that regulates wake-sleep cycles, and causes drowsiness. Some people are sensitive to even small amounts of caffeine, and can experience jitters, anxiety and nervousness, rapid heartbeat, and insomnia. Caffeine-free coffee and tea are readily available,

although not every trace of caffeine may be removed.
- **Salicylates** are found naturally in plant-based foods, and serve to help protect the plants from environmental incursions. Foods that have higher than average salicylates include vegetables, fruits, coffee, tea, nuts, spices, and honey, and generally are tolerated by most people, and some studies suggest that salicylates may help prevent colorectal cancer. But a small percentage of people are sensitive to even small amounts of salicylates, and develop respiratory symptoms, like stuffy nose, asthma, nasal and sinus polyps, as well as diarrhea, and hives. Since it's not possible to completely remove salicylates from foods, those who have salicylate intolerance should avoid spices, raisins, oranges, and coffee, and any other foods they may find they are sensitive to. They should also be alert to medication and cosmetics that contain salicylates as preservatives.
- **Histamines** are a compound that is produced naturally in foods and in our bodies, and plays a valuable role in the immune system, and the digestive and nervous systems. Histamines help protect us from infection by initiating immediate inflammatory responses to allergens, often leading to sneezing, watery eyes, and itching to excrete harmful invaders. Most people metabolize histamines, but those who

are unable to effectively break down, metabolize, and excrete it may experience symptoms like hives, itching, and stomach cramps. They should avoid high-histamine-containing foods which tend to be fermented, preserved, smoked (like fish), cured (like meats), dried, soured (like buttermilk), citrus fruits, and avocados.

- **FODMAPs** are fermentable oligo-saccharides, di-saccharides, mono-saccharides and polyols, which are short-chain carbohydrates in many foods that can cause digestive distress. FODMAPs are not well absorbed in the small intestine, so their nutrients are not digested, and travel to the colon, where they become prebiotics to feed the lower gut bacteria. We'll come back to FODMAPs in great depth and detail starting in chapter 5.
- **Sulfites** can be found naturally in some foods, and are often used as preservatives. Those who are hypersensitive to sulfites can experience symptoms like wheezing, stuffy nose, and low blood pressure. Be alert to sulfites used to keep the color in dried fruits, and in wine, apple cider, vinegar, canned and pickled foods. In extreme cases, in addition to the usual reactions, plus hives, swelling, and diarrhea, sulfites can cause constriction of the airways, which can be life-threatening. The FDA requires that the

addition or possible presence of sulfites from processing, be listed on packaging.

Other causes of food intolerances include:

- **Aspartame** is an artificial sweetener used as a sugar substitute. Some studies have shown side effects including irritability and depression among those with sensitivity.
- **Eggs** may cause sensitivity among people who have difficulty digesting egg whites, but are not otherwise allergic to eggs. Symptoms include diarrhea and abdominal pain.
- **Food colorings** like Red 40 and Yellow 5 have been found to cause sensitivity reactions in some. Symptoms may include skin swelling, hives, and stuffy nose.
- **Yeast intolerance** usually causes less severe symptoms than yeast allergies. Symptoms are normally limited to the digestive system and include bloating, gas, diarrhea, and nausea.
- **Sugar alcohols** may be used as calorie-free sugar alternatives. They may cause digestive problems in sensitive people, including bloating and diarrhea.

Hepatitis and Gallstones

We'll conclude this chapter with two conditions that are outside the GI tract, but very much part of the overall digestive system, by affecting the liver and the gallbladder.

But now a quick review from the first chapter. The liver is an essential organ that processes nutrients, and fights infections. The liver's functions include production and secretion of bile, and cleansing the blood arriving from the small intestine. The bile passes from the liver through a passageway, the cystic duct, into a small, pear-shaped organ, the gallbladder where it is stored. When food arrives in the small intestine, contractions of the gallbladder deliver bile to aid in the nutrient separations. Bile, you will recall, is a yellowish-green brown syrupy liquid that is delivered from the gallbladder to the duodenum section of the small intestine to aid in the breaking down of fats, leading to more effective digestion and absorption. Bile also helps increase the contractions of peristalsis.

Given the importance of these two organs, any diseases that affect them can be of considerable concern.

Hepatitis

Hepatitis is defined as an inflammation of the liver. Depending on the cause and type, the disease may be self-limiting, or it can advance to more serious conditions: fibrosis, or scarring, cirrhosis, or it may progress to liver cancer. The most common causes of hepatitis worldwide are hepatitis viruses, but other types of infections, trauma from toxic substances like alcohol, or some drugs, and autoimmune diseases may also cause hepatitis. The most common forms of viral hepatitis in the U.S. are the well-known hepatitis A, B, and C:

- **Hepatitis A** is the least serious form. It is often contracted from eating food infected with contaminated fecal matter, and lasts from a few weeks, to a few months, in most cases. Hepatitis A can be prevented by vaccine, which is recommended for children, and those who travel internationally. About 24,900 new cases are diagnosed annually in the U.S.
- **Hepatitis B** is a more serious form of the disease, and is spread primarily through person-to-person contact and exchange of bodily fluid, including semen and blood, or other fluids in microscopic amounts. The virus travels from someone infected with the hepatitis B virus to someone who is uninfected. The hepatitis B virus may be transmitted from sexual relations, sharing contaminated syringes, or even razors or toothbrushes if traces of blood are present. An infant can be infected by the mother during birth. Up to 25% of people who are chronically infected may develop chronic liver diseases, like liver failure, cirrhosis (scarring of the liver), or even liver cancer. A preventative vaccine is available, and recommended for those at risk of exposure, including drug users, and those who

live with, or work with, infected persons. About 22,600 new cases occur each year in the U.S., and about 900,000 are living with the disease.
- **Hepatitis C** is the most serious form of this disease. Up to 50% of those who are exposed develop a long-term chronic infection, and from 5% to 25% develop cirrhosis over 10 to 20 years. It may be spread in the same manner as hepatitis B, although bodily fluids are limited to blood, albeit even the smallest quantities can be infectious, as from a shared syringe, for example. Prior to 1992 it could be passed by transfusion, but blood and plasma screenings now prevent that possibility. There are 50,000 new cases of Hepatitis C in the U.S. annually, and 2.4 million are infected.

Hepatitis A is generally treated with supportive care, and efforts to prevent further infection. Hepatitis B in acute form is also treated with supportive care, since there is no specific cure. If the disease is chronic, antiviral drugs may be prescribed as part of the treatment.

Chronic hepatitis C infections are now able to be treated effectively, and in a short time. Medicine has made considerable progress in treating chronic hepatitis C with new antiviral medications which are direct acting, and may supplement other medications. Good outcomes with fewer side effects may be experienced within eight weeks. Medications are tailored to each individual, based on the extent of liver damage, the disease genotype, previous treatments, and other conditions. There is a 90% cure rate, but in extreme, advanced cases of liver damage, a liver transplant may be required.

Any form of hepatitis can be a hidden disease, with many of those who are infected having few or no symptoms, and they can be unaware of their infection. If an acute infection manifests itself, it may do so from two weeks to six months after they have been exposed. Chronic viral hepatitis symptoms may remain dormant for years or even decades. Chronic symptoms may include loss of appetite, fatigue, fever, abdominal pain, nausea and vomiting, joint pain, light-colored stool, and dark urine. Jaundice, which is yellowing of the skin, is a classic characteristic of chronic hepatitis infection. Doctors use blood tests primarily to diagnose hepatitis, but additional evaluations may be made by CT scan and MRI examinations of the liver.

Gallstones

Small, hard deposits can form in the gallbladder, most often as an accumulation of cholesterol. According to *Harvard Health Publishing* (2011), 80% of gallstones are formed by cholesterol, with the remaining 20% being buildups of bilirubin and calcium salts. Cholesterol stones form when there is an excess of cholesterol in the liver; bilirubin stones are dark brown in color, due to their being the end result of old blood cells that are destroyed by the liver. When there is an excess of bilirubin accumulating in the gallbladder that can't be broken down, the stones form. Regardless of the source, stones are likely to form when the gallbladder does not empty its bile with sufficient regularity or completeness.

Gallstones affect 25 million people in the U.S., with the majority being women: 65% to 75%. In most cases, gallstones may not cause serious symptoms, and when there are problems, they can be resolved.

Symptoms include pain in the upper right abdomen, often brought on from eating fried or greasy foods, and lasting for a few hours. Other symptoms may include nausea and vomiting, dark urine, clay colored stools, abdominal pain, burping, indigestion, and diarrhea. Gallstones do not cause pain; rather, pain occurs when the flow of bile is blocked from exiting the gallbladder. Since 80% of cases are asymptomatic, doctors may only discover the presence of gallstones from X-rays for other purposes or during abdominal surgery.

In rare cases (1% to 3%), the bile may become completely blocked by the gallstones, causing a medical emergency called acute cholecystitis. Symptoms include extreme pain in the upper abdomen or upper-right back, fever, and chills.

Risk factors apart from gender (female), age (60+), or having a family history of gallstones, include being overweight or obese, having a diet rich in cholesterol or fat, or low in fiber, have sudden weight loss, or have diabetes mellitus. Persons of Native American and Mexican-American descent are also of higher risk, and should be attentive to controllable factors, like weight and diet.

Diagnosis after symptoms have been reported, can be through ultrasound, (the preferred technique), abdominal CT scan, a gallbladder radionuclide scan, or blood tests to measure levels of bilirubin in the blood.

Treatment for gallstones is often not needed unless the person is in pain, and they may pass naturally, without the person being aware. If there is pain, surgery to remove the gallstones may be necessary. An alternative to surgery is placement of a drainage tube through the skin. Medications may be prescribed in rare cases.

The following chapter is devoted to a single chronic gastrointestinal disorder, known as leaky gut.

Chapter 4:

Is Your Gut Leaking?

Leaky gut? Really? Can your gut actually leak, and if so, what it is leaking, and where is it leaking to?

Evidence is mounting to verify that yes, your gut can indeed leak, as a result of certain foods in your diet that are not being digested in the correct section of your GI tract, and as a result, microbe, toxins, and fluids that should remain securely in your gut are slipping through barriers to enter the bloodstream and go to parts of your body where they don't belong. At the same time, nutrients that your body needs are not being fully absorbed and sent to cells and organs where needed; all in all, it's a lose-lose situation, and many people who may have a leaky gut are not aware of it, or the problems it causes. Or so the theory goes. But is it based on solid science?

Is leaky gut syndrome a real medical condition, and can it lead to autoimmune disorders and chronic diseases if it is not recognized and treated? Gastroenterologists are approaching leaky gut with increasing interest, given the growing evidence, but some are still hesitant to give it full acknowledgement and recognition, in part because many of its symptoms can be attributed to other diseases and conditions. Consider how many diseases you read about in the previous chapter, including IBS and IBD, among many others, that have symptoms like abdominal pain, sensitivity to certain foods, nausea and vomiting, unexplained weight loss, fever, chills, diarrhea, and hives; some of these same symptoms may also be attributed to leaky gut, as you will see. Is leaky gut being blamed for symptoms that should be attributable to other diseases?

There is still some skepticism in the medical field about whether it really exists, but fortunately, leaky gut syndrome is no longer flying under the radar. It is being recognized by a widening circle of gastroenterologists and nutritionists, and dietary solutions are being developed. The following chapters are devoted to the FODMAP diet, which is believed to be able to resolve leaky gut, and many other food-induced disorders, but first, let's get to know leaky gut and all of its characteristics, and the problems it creates.

Based on the research and science you are about to read, you can decide just how real leaky gut syndrome is, and whether it's affecting you. The first section gathers the evidence, and the second section explores the full range of conditions leaky gut can cause.

How Real Is Leaky Gut?

According to Donald Kirby MD, gastroenterologist, and director of the Cleveland Clinic's Center for Human Nutrition, leaky gut syndrome is a very gray area. He explains, "Physicians don't know enough about the gut, which is our biggest immune system organ." Leaky gut syndrome is not taught in medical school, so it is not part of the gastroenterologists' or internists' standard catalog of GI tract diseases, and so diagnosis of its symptoms can be challenging, and hard to differentiate from other diseases.

Gastroenterologist Linda A. Lee, MD, director of Johns Hopkins Integrative Medicine and Digestive Center says, "In the absence of evidence, we don't know what it (leaky gut) means or what therapies can directly address it."

So what is leaky gut syndrome, or at least, what do the professionals think it is?

Leaky gut is believed to be a condition that allows bacteria and toxins to exit the GI tract, especially through the walls of the small intestine. The leading explanation for the "leak" is increased intestinal permeability, or hyperpermeability. There are tight, tiny junctions in the small intestine, which normally allow nutrients and water to enter the bloodstream by passing through the intestinal lining. If those very small openings are somehow enlarged or opened wider, bacteria and toxic substances could leak into the bloodstream, leading to inflammation and immune system responses.

Hyperpermeability is already recognized medically, and is believed to be caused by celiac disease and Crohn's disease, making it harder to attribute the phenomenon to yet another disorder, leaky gut syndrome. Dr. Lee acknowledges that different, yet unconfirmed diseases may be at work, saying, "We don't know all the causes," and she questions whether hyperpermeability is a contributing factor on its own, or is a consequence of other conditions.

These uncertainties are why many mainstream medical professionals do not yet recognize leaky gut syndrome as a unique and distinctive condition. Some dismiss leaky gut as taking "credit" for symptoms of other, well-known diseases, and believe it is not a distinctive disease, but simply an umbrella description of hyperpermeability caused by other diseases and conditions.

Yet believers in leaky gut are tenacious in their convictions, claiming that it's a distinct disease, and can be the underlying cause of numerous conditions, like migraine headaches, food sensitivities, chronic fatigue syndrome, fibromyalgia, thyroid abnormalities, multiple sclerosis, mood swings, skin conditions and even autism, and other Asperger's spectrum disorders.

According to John's Hopkins' Dr. Lee, some doctors do not bother to work to get at the true cause of the symptoms, and that can often drive patients to practitioners of alternative medicine. Lee says, "We need to listen," and combines complementary therapies that are based on evidence, with conventional medicine in her clinic. The evidence associated with leaky gut, what causes it and how to effectively treat it has been slow to accumulate. This is something that is essential for patients to understand.

Lee says "We are in the infancy of understanding what to do," and is concerned that some marketers who are making claims about effective treatment are doing so without supportive evidence. She cites websites that are recommending L-glutamine supplements, claiming that the nutrients will reinforce and strengthen the small intestinal lining, despite there being no scientific or clinical proof to substantiate such claims. "There's no evidence that if I give you a pile of glutamine pills, that you will improve," Lee says. The best option for doctors is to diagnose a "probable" known underlying condition, like IBS, especially Crohn's disease, and recommend recognized treatments.

As with IBS and IBD, diet probably plays an important, perhaps decisive role in causing or exacerbating leaky gut, a perspective on which doctors Lee and Kirby concur. A person who shows symptoms of leaky gut should see a nutrition-trained gastroenterologist.

Author's note: *After I experienced certain lower GI tract symptoms, my gastroenterologist introduced me to the FODMAP diet, which was helpful in identifying foods that probably needed to be avoided, while allowing me to resume many other foods and beverages which proved to be asymptomatic.* - J.E.

Stress is also a possible cause of leaky gut, since chronic stress can cause immune responses that lead to inflammation, which, in turn, can create imbalances in the gut. Stress can cause the central nervous system to activate the fight-or-flight sympathetic nervous system response, which causes the action hormones adrenaline and cortisol to increase glucose in the blood, which raises heart and breathing rates, elevates blood pressure, and, of significance, interrupts the digestive process. Managing stress can help reduce the symptoms of leaky gut, so introduction of stress-reducing activities and behavior into the lifestyle, like yoga, meditation, and exercise, are recommended.

What Are the Causes?

Leaky gut syndrome remains a pretty much a mystery among medical professionals who are still trying to understand precisely what causes it. There is one suspect at this time, Zonulin, which is a protein that is the only recognized regulator of intestinal permeability.

When Zonulin is activated in people who are genetically susceptible, it can initiate a conduction of intestinal permeability that has the appearance of the condition created by leaky gut. Zonulin can be released by certain strains of intestinal bacteria and by ingestion of gluten, which, as you know from the earlier description, is a protein in wheat, rye, spelt, and some other grains. But other research has shown that gluten's effect on intestinal permeability is limited to conditions like celiac disease, irritable bowel syndrome, and other bowel disorders.

A multitude of factors can contribute to leaky gut syndrome. In addition to the already mentioned roles of long-term stress and chronic inflammation, these are commonly cited as possible causes:

- Excessive sugar in the diet, especially fructose, is unhealthy and can disrupt the intestinal wall's barrier function. Sugar is abundant today in prepared foods, soft drinks, sports beverages

and energy drinks, as well as in the customary desserts and snacks.
- NSAIDs, or non-steroidal anti-inflammatory drugs, which are common OTC pain relievers and fever reducers like ibuprofen, aspirin and naproxen can increase intestinal permeability and contribute to leaky gut, when used frequently over the long-term.
- Excessive alcohol consumption can increase intestinal permeability. Most health authorities recommend no more than one drink per day for women, and a limit of two for men.
- Deficiencies in vitamins A and D, zinc, and other minerals have each been suspected of contributing to increased intestinal permeability.
- Imbalances in the microbiome can cause poor gut health, especially when the non beneficial bacteria become abundant. Some strains of bacteria can weaken the intestinal wall's barrier function, leading to permeability.
- Yeast is naturally found in the GI tract, including the intestines, but if conditions cause the yeast cells to proliferate and become overabundant, the overgrowth might contribute to leaky gut.

Yet, many professionals are not so sure that all of these factors are legitimate "smoking guns," or highly likely causes of leaky gut, or any other type of hyperpermeability. According to Aparajita Singh, M.D., who is a gastroenterologist and associate professor of gastroenterology at the University of California San Francisco, "I've never told a patient, 'You have leaky gut syndrome,' but I've heard it many times."

Leaky Gut and You

Leaky gut: what it is, how it manifests itself, its symptoms, and what it means for gut health.

Leaky Gut-Caused Diseases

In addition to being a disease in its own right, leaky gut can set you up to be susceptible to other diseases. Online publications and other sources of health news and advice suggest that leaky gut syndrome might be associated with everything from nutritional deficiencies and food allergies to fatigue, joint pain, and autoimmune disorders. Let's get a closer look through the perspectives of competent medical authorities.

The concept of leaky gut syndrome is founded on the existence in the gut of intestinal permeability, which is still becoming understood, and is the subject of some controversy among doctors. Your GI tract contains particles of food, bacteria and other microbes, like viruses, and toxins, keeping them inside the intestines, and from entering the bloodstream. Managing what stays within the intestines, and what can safely pass is the intestinal membrane, which you will recall is lined with strands of villi, that allow only nutrients and water to pass into the bloodstream. According to UCSF's Dr. Singh, having a weakened intestinal barrier enables potentially harmful bacteria and toxins to leak out, and potentially lead to diseases and symptoms.

Our understanding of how the intestinal barrier functions has evolved in recent years. Previously, it was believed that the intestinal lining's cells are somehow connected by tight intersections, or junctions, described as, "Tight junctions like mortar between two bricks," according to the Cleveland Clinic's Dr. Kirby. But today, doctors are now recognizing that the tight junctions, "Are more like canals, and they can open and close. So they can, under certain circumstances, get a little weaker," he says.

There is normally a base level of permeability in the membrane to permit the flow of nutrients, electrolytes, and water from the small intestine into the bloodstream. However, it has been observed that the junctions are looser in those who have received chemotherapy treatment for cancer, Dr. Kirby notes. Then there is the balance of bacteria naturally in the gut, which can potentially play a role in permeability, according to Dr. Felice Schnoll-Sussman, director of the Jay Monahan Center for Gastrointestinal Health at NewYork-Presbyterian and Weill Cornell Medicine. There is some observational evidence that diet, including consumption of processed foods, alcohol, and caffeine, as well as use of NSAIDs, could increase the permeability of the membrane, says Dr. Singh. But for now, these have not been verified in clinical trials, and so these are just theories for now.

Building Your Gut Health

What can you do to avoid leaky gut, or reduce its symptoms if you have them? Since leaky gut syndrome does not have official medical recognition as a disease, there is currently no recommended treatment. Of course, your doctor or gastroenterologist may decide your symptoms point to one of the IBS or IBD diseases, and prescribe appropriate medications, and dietary recommendations. One of those recommendations might be the FODMAP diet, if food sensitivities are suspected.

Dr. Marcelo Campos, commenting on leaky gut syndrome in *Harvard Health Publishing* (2017), says that your DNA, or inherited propensities, may not be to blame for the symptom of leaky gut. He suggests that modern life can be a primary driver of gut inflammation and similar conditions. He cites a rising tide of evidence that the typical American diet, which tends to be high in sugar and saturated fats, while being low in dietary fiber, may be the catalyst of inflammation and other GI tract imbalances, perhaps leading to conditions favorable to leaky gut. In addition, Dr. Campos thinks that stress, and overindulgence in alcohol, may also contribute to the imbalances.

The Dietary Solution

Dr. Campos leads us to the obvious conclusion: you may be able to reduce or eliminate symptoms of leaky gut and improve your overall digestive health, by following a diet rich in the kinds of foods that support the growth of gut bacteria that are beneficial. Your objective is to favor and nurture the good bacteria, while diminishing the unhealthy gut bacteria that have been linked to negative health outcomes, like chronic inflammation from an overactive immune system. A healthy diet can help protect you as well from various types of cancer, heart disease, and type 2 diabetes, so what's to lose? If you will be following the FODMAP diet, you should be able to include many of these foods, even during the first, elimination phase.

As a general rule, a diet that supports digestive health should be based on natural, unprocessed foods that do not contain added sugar, are low in salt (sodium), and include fibrous vegetables and fermented vegetables, as well as fruits, cultured dairy products, healthy oils and fats, and lean meats. These foods are the basis of what is called the Mediterranean diet, and provides great options for improving your digestive health, while enjoying what you eat:

- Vegetables, including broccoli, kale, cabbage, arugula, Brussels sprouts, carrots, beets, Swiss chard, spinach, mushrooms, zucchini, and virtually all leafy vegetables. Select from a diversity of colors (like red, green yellow, purple) to obtain different vitamins and minerals.
- Potatoes and sweet potatoes, winter squash, and turnips. Don't peel potatoes to retain the valuable fiber.
- Fermented vegetables, which are probiotic, and can include sauerkraut, pickles, tempeh, kimchi,

and miso. (Be careful not to cook fermented foods, to avoid killing the live bacteria.)
- Most fresh fruits and berries, including blueberries, grapes, strawberries, bananas, kiwis, raspberries, pineapple, oranges, papaya, mangos, and passionfruit. As with vegetables, it's good to have a diversity of colors.
- Dried fruits are also rich in nutrients, and include prunes, raisins, dates, figs, sliced mangos, and apricots. Look for versions that are not preserved with sulfites, and be careful with quantities, because dried fruits are high in calories, due to density.
- Sprouted and unsprouted seeds, including chia seeds, flax seeds, sunflower seeds, and hemp seeds.
- Gluten-free grains, including buckwheat, rice (brown), amaranth, sorghum, teff, and gluten-free oats. Select whole grains to benefit from the nutrients and fiber in the outer husk. If you like to bake, you can use whole grain flours milled from these gluten-free grains.
- Healthy fats from whole avocados, and from monounsaturated avocado oil, and extra virgin olive oil, and secondarily, polyunsaturated soybean, sunflower, corn, and safflower oils. Unsaturated oils are liquid at room temperature.
- Fish is an excellent source of complete protein as well as antioxidants and other nutrients.

Choose cold-water salmon, tuna, herring, mackerel, sardines, and other omega-3-rich fish.
- Meats are also an excellent source of complete protein, but your selection should be limited to lean cuts of moderate-sized portions of chicken, turkey, beef, lamb, and pork.
- Eggs are again recognized as a nutritionally valuable part of a healthy diet. One egg per day is an excellent source of complete protein, with low fat, and other nutrients. Cardiologists are now okay with the cholesterol in eggs, as long as a limit of 7 per week is observed.
- Herbs and spices; just about all have trace minerals and other nutrients.
- Low-fat and nonfat milk and other dairy products are an excellent source of protein; cultured dairy contains probiotic bacteria, and includes yogurt (especially higher protein Greek and Icelandic-style yogurts), cottage cheese, buttermilk, and kefir.
- Beverages of benefit, apart from milk, include coffee (up to four cups a day are considered okay), black and green teas (green is lower in caffeine), milk-style beverages made from coconuts, almonds, oats, rice, and soya. Of course, water is abundant, calorie-free, and essential.
- Nuts, both raw and dry roasted, including walnuts, pecans, peanuts, and almonds are high in protein and beneficial oils. Peanut butter (and

butter made from other nuts) is high in nutritional benefits, if it is minimally processed, and contains only ground nuts, and no added sugar, fats, or preservatives. Be aware that nuts and nut products are high in calories due to the oil content.

The other side of the nutritional equation is the list of foods that not only can have negative effects on your digestive health, but are mostly to avoid for good cardiovascular health, better weight management, and prevention of diabetes, and other diseases. Despite any initial disappoint in giving up certain foods you like, you will discover a new satisfaction with more natural, non greasy, health-giving, wholesome foods, and your gut will thank you.

- Grains and cereals containing gluten: wheat, rye, barley, and triticale. This includes products made with wheat, especially: bread, pasta, couscous, and most cereals. Note: If the FODMAP diet shows that you have no sensitivity to wheat, you may not have to avoid foods containing gluten. Despite the public interest in gluten-free products, most people do not have sensitivity to gluten, as discussed earlier.
- Processed meats, including bacon, cold cuts, frankfurters, sausages, salami, bologna, and other deli meats. Stick with natural, unprocessed lean meats.

- Baked goods that are high in sugar and saturated fats, including most types of cakes and muffins, pies, cookies, and most pastries. Doughnuts are high in fats and sugar, and are definitely to be avoided.
- Snack foods that are high in sugars and saturated fats, and that are made with refined wheat. Read the labels, and go for snacks that are made without sugar, and limited to simple, natural ingredients like nuts and dried fruits.
- Junk food is a blanket term that is applied to greasy, high fat or sugary foods, including most candy bars, potato chips, and presweetened cereals. Exception: chocolate is considered healthful, and can be part of your diet if it is at least 70% cacao (85% is better, once you get used to it).
- What about pizza, America's favorite meal (it replaced the hamburger in popularity years ago)? Most pizza made with wheat has to be avoided, but there are pizza crusts being made from alternatives, including gluten-free cauliflower. For health, avoid heavy cheese toppings, and be alert to high sodium levels in the sauce and crust. Skip toppings like pepperoni and other preserved meats.
- Artificial sweeteners, like aspartame, sucralose, and saccharin are not beneficial, even if they replace sugar in your diet. Your gut gets confused by these products and sends mixed

signals to your brain, including unnecessary appetite stimulation.
- Sauces like soy, teriyaki, and hoisin are very high in sodium and should be avoided or used very sparingly. Most salad dressings are loaded with oils and may contain salt or sugar, or both. Check labels for simple, natural dressings or better, make your own with extra virgin olive oil and balsamic vinegar. Mix in some yogurt for a creamy dressing.
- Beverages that contain sugar are to be avoided, including soft drinks, sports beverages, and energy drinks. If you drink alcohol, do so in moderation: one drink per day for women; two at most for men. One drink means 5 oz wine, 1.5 oz spirits, or one 12 oz bottle or can of beer. If you don't drink alcohol, it's best not to start.

Concerns about excessive alcohol consumption leads us back to Dr. Campos, who also included stress as one of the risk factors for the onset of leaky gut symptoms. Let's give your lifestyle some attention.

Lifestyle Stress Management

We experience stress because our bodies evolved to survive during times when we are in danger. Our reaction has been finely tuned through the ages so we can switch into high gear within mere seconds to escape fires, floods, famine, and hostile encounters. These survival instincts remain with us, and can be activated easily by any sudden concern. If the surge of energy, and elevated cardiovascular and respiratory responses are temporary, and subside as soon as the risks are gone; no problem, the body goes back to normal. But when we allow ourselves to remain ready for action on a continuing basis, when everything bothers us, it becomes chronic stress, and our defensive reactions continue over time. This leads to inflammation, which leads to more immune responses. And one of the casualties of this situation is our gastrointestinal system.

Why? Because when the fight-or-flight response is underway, a signal goes from our brain stem through the vagus nerve to the digestive system, and tells it to shut down, so the body can divert energy to the muscles. This means the process of peristalsis, which are the contractions that move food through the gut, stops. Everything stops. Food stays in the stomach, and in the small and large intestine. In the intestines, the bacteria in the microbiome are confused. Digestive acids accumulate without enough food to absorb them, and a buildup of toxins occurs. Damage to the walls of the small intestine is inevitable.

Does this all lead to a leaky gut? No one is positive yet, but it looks probable, and worth the effort to get out from under the injuries from chronic stress. These are easy and accessible solutions. We've mentioned these options before, and they're worth repeating. Practice any one, or preferably, all three:

With just 20 to 30 minutes, a series of yoga stretches and poses can bring down the stress, and put you into a state of calm. You can learn downward dog, warrior, child's pose, cat cow, and the other beginner poses from a wide range of videos online, or you can join a yoga class and benefit from the instructor's guidance. You will also learn the stress-lowering benefits of managed breathing, and how to focus your concentration. Unless you've had previous training, start at the beginner level, and be patient if you feel a little stiff and unbalanced to start.

It's been many decades since the Beatles introduced the Westen world to transcendental meditation, but today, in its many forms, meditation is more popular than ever, due largely to its verified stress-reduction qualities. In summary, meditation is a state of concentration that prevents distractions from outside, intruding thoughts. This singular focus has been proven clinically to lower tension, stress, and anxiety, as well as help reduce depression. As with yoga, managed breathing is an essential part of the procedure. It takes from 10 to 20 minutes to achieve the relaxation response, and can be practiced anywhere you can sit comfortably and not be disturbed. There are many instructive videos online, and there are apps you can download that provide guidance through the meditation, with calming voices and restful background sounds and music.

You are probably aware of the importance of physical exercise to help lower the risks of heart disease, obesity, diabetes, even cancer, and many other diseases, but exercise is equally valuable in reducing chronic stress, and the inflammation and immune disorders it induces. It can also provide calm during brief situations of stress and anxiety, and can help alleviate depression. Consider adopting a cardiovascular conditioning routine, with your choice of jogging, brisk walking, swimming, or using an elliptical machine or stationary cycle. A total of

150 minutes per week of moderate exercise, or 75 minutes of fast paced cardio exercise is recommended.

- Add two or three days when you perform resistance exercises to further reduce stress, while building lean muscle. If you do not have access to a gym or fitness center for weightlifting, you can perform bodyweight calisthenics at home with little or no equipment. There are many excellent demonstration videos for calisthenics online.

Whether you will be trying to practice yoga, or engage in exercise, always be sure to ease into it gradually, to avoid discomfort and possible injury. It's more beneficial to do some light stretching, without forcing the movements, for about 10 minutes before starting yoga, cardio, or resistance exercises. Then, if you are going to do yoga or resistance, it's a good idea to start with 10 to 15 minutes of cardio, to really get the muscles warmed up and the blood flowing. Okay, you are ready to begin learning all about the FODMAP diet, and what it can do for your gastrointestinal health.

Chapter 5:

Is FODMAP Diet the Answer?

Whether your concern is irritable bowel syndrome, or inflammatory bowel diseases like Crohn's disease or ulcerative colitis, or possibly you, or someone you know, suspects a case of leaky gut, most gastroenterologists try to resolve the problem through diet. And the diet that is getting more and more attention now is the FODMAP diet, and its process of elimination and restoration of foods that are determined to be safe.

As you have already seen, most of those diseases and syndromes have similar symptoms, making it hard for doctors to precisely identify which of those diseases a person may be suffering from. However, because the FODMAP diet can be effective in identifying dietary components that are potentially the causes of the diseases, it can serve to resolve the symptoms of each disease.

This chapter covers the basics of the FODMAP diet, its connection to the health of the GI tract, and it's potential ability to effectively cure digestive system disorders.

What are FODMAP Foods?

FODMAP is the acronym or abbreviation for "Fermentable Oligosaccharides, Disaccharides, Monosaccharides, And Polyols." Quite a mouthful, so to speak, so let's break this down into manageable language.

The foods we eat are classified with three major food groups: carbohydrates, proteins, and fat. In summary:

Carbohydrates are the largest component of our diet, providing energy to every cell, every muscle fiber, and every organ. Familiar sources of carbohydrates in our diet include fruits and vegetables, grains and cereals, nuts and seeds, beans, lentils and other legumes, and dairy products, like milk and yogurt. But these foods may also be sources of the other two food groups. Pure carbohydrates are represented by sugar, honey, agave and corn syrups, and alcohol. Carbohydrates are built up of simple molecules called saccharides.

Protein is the building block of our bodies, and provides the structure of our muscles, organs, hormones, enzymes, and every one of the trillions of cells in our bodies. Dietary protein is in its most concentrated form in meat and fish and other animal-sourced foods, like milk, cheese, yogurt, and other dairy products, plus the white of eggs. But proteins are also found, in secondary quantities, in many vegetables, grains and cereals, beans and lentils, nuts and seeds. Vegetarians and vegans are able to obtain adequate quantities of protein by eating a variety of plant sources.

Proteins are built up of complex molecules called amino acids.

Fats are also used in bodies for energy, but unlike carbohydrates, they are primarily used for storage of energy, rather than for more immediate needs, like carbohydrates. Dietary fats are provided by meat and dairy products, but fats from those sources tend to be high in unhealthy saturated fats, which can lead to heart disease, so fats from nuts and seeds, vegetables, grains and cereals, are preferable. These healthier monounsaturated and polyunsaturated fats are liquid at room temperature and are called oils. Fats and oils are composed of fatty acids, and contain nine calories per gram, compared to four calories per gram for carbohydrates and proteins.

Carbohydrates: The Basics

FODMAP foods are all short chain carbohydrates, so we should begin by understanding what that means: carbohydrates are organic compounds (in chemistry, organic means based on carbon, and is not related to organic foods). In addition to carbon, they are composed of hydrogen, and oxygen, often in a 1:2:1 ratio. These three elements give rise to the name, carbohydrates, and they are one of the major classes of biomolecules. Carbohydrates are an essential food source of energy, and also serve as structural components, such as fiber (imagine a stalk of celery). As nutrients, they are classified as either simple carbohydrates, or as complex carbohydrates:

- Simple carbohydrates, also known simply as sugars, are readily digested, and can provide an

immediate source of energy. But a potential downside of simple carbohydrates in our diet are blood sugar spikes.
- Complex carbohydrates are also known as saccharide polymers, and are slower to digest and to metabolize. Complex carbohydrates include starches, they tend to be high in fiber, and because of their complexity, are not likely to cause blood sugar spikes.

Saccharides and Polyols

This brings us to the components of FODMAPs. Carbohydrates are built up from individual unit molecular structures called saccharides:

- **Monosaccharide**, the most simple, is a molecule made of only one saccharide unit.
- **Disaccharide,** is a larger molecule, and as the name implies, is made of two saccharide units.
- **Oligosaccharide** means "few saccharides," and is composed typically of three to ten smaller monosaccharide molecular units.

These three types of saccharides are represented by the O, D, and M in FODMAP. Here are the remaining components, F, A (for And), and P, and their meaning:

- **Fermentable** means these saccharides are capable of being fermented in the large intestine, by bacteria in the microbiome. It's the fermentation, in the wrong part of the GI tract,

that is believed to be the cause of many digestive disorders.
- **Polyols** refers to certain carbohydrates that are found in some fruits and vegetables, or that can be synthesized for use as food additives, for sweetness. They are also called sugar alcohols, and are designated as a FODMAP food that can irritate the gut because they are slow to absorb, and ferment rapidly in the large intestine. Some polyols are as sweet as sugar and may be added to artificial sweaters, like aspartame.

Once again, here is FODMAP in the proper sequence: "Fermentable Oligosaccharides, Disaccharides, Monosaccharides, and Polyols."

To give you an idea of how monosaccharides can combine to form more complex carbohydrates, common granulated table sugar is actually a disaccharide, called sucrose, composed of a glucose monosaccharide and a fructose monosaccharide. Other disaccharides include maltose (two glucose monosaccharides), and lactose, or milk sugar (one glucose and one galactose monosaccharide). When two monosaccharides combine to form a disaccharide, the process is called dehydration, because a water molecule (H_2O) is released; conversely, hydrolysis, the capturing of a water molecule occurs, when two monosaccharides are separated, as during digestion, for example.

One of the primary sources of glucose in nature is photosynthesis in plants, where it is stored as energy. Fructose is also produced in plants, especially fruits (which is why it may be referred to as fruit sugar), and combines with glucose to form sucrose for efficient energy storage in plants.

Glucose and fructose are also present in honey, as the result of more complex sucrose disaccharides being digested and broken down in the stomachs of bees into monosaccharides.

This is the same as when we ingest sucrose, and an enzyme in our small intestine, invertase, breaks it back into its component glucose and fructose monosaccharide components. Glucose is then converted to glycogen and stored in our muscles for energy when needed. The fructose, however, is not so easily stored or put to beneficial use, and may end up in the large intestine, where the FODMAP problems occur.

How Can FODMAP Foods Affect You?

Sensitivity to FODMAP foods varies by individual; reactions to FODMAPs can range from none, with complete digestion accomplished in the small intestine, to intense reaction and severe symptoms. In most cases of FODMAPs sensitivity, a limited group of foods may be the cause of the problem, and once these specific foods are eliminated from the diet, the symptoms subside or completely disappear.

Impact on Your Microbiome

FODMAPs are short-chain carbohydrates that can be resistant to digestion, depending on each individual's digestive system. In certain instances, instead of being digested in the small intestine and absorbed into your bloodstream, these carbohydrates reach the large intestine (the colon), where most of your gut bacteria reside. These bacteria then use these carbohydrates for fuel, causing digestive symptoms.

Good, or friendly bacteria generally produce methane gas, while the types of microbiome bacteria that favor feeding on FODMAPs generate hydrogen gas, which can cause intestinal gas and bloating, stomach cramps and intestinal pain, and constipation, as well as a distended stomach. In addition, the bacterial processing of FODMAPs can attract water into your large intestine, an effect called being osmotically active, and instead of constipation, can lead to diarrhea.

An example of the action of FODMAP foods in the GI tract is the accumulation of undigested fructose that is malabsorbed in the small intestine, and subsequently transported to the large intestine. There, certain strains of microbiome bacteria may cause fermentation of the fructose monosaccharides, resulting in symptoms like those of IBD, leaky gut, and IBS, including diarrhea, gas and bloating, cramps and abdominal pain.

Foods High in FODMAPs

The following chapter will provide extensive listings of foods and their degree of FODMAP sensitivity, but in overview, most FODMAP foods fall into these categories:

- Fructose, or fruit sugar, is a monosaccharide occurring in many vegetables and fruits. It is combined with glucose to make sucrose, or common sugar, and in the gut, digestive fluids can separate sucrose back into the two monosaccharides. Fruits that are high-FODMAP include apples and pears, figs, cherries, apricots, mangoes, plums, nectarines and peaches, and watermelon. Interestingly, other fruits—from bananas and blueberries to papayas, pineapples and strawberries—are low-FODMAP.
- Lactose is a disaccharide found in dairy products, especially milk. Many people are lactose intolerant and have an option to use lactose-free milk, allowing them to continue drinking milk during all phases of the FODMAP diet.
- Fructans are in certain grains, especially wheat, rye, barley, and spelt. Fructans are not related to gluten, which is actually a protein, and is rated low on the FODMAP list of foods. Wheat is of concern because of the quantity consumed; in small quantities it too is rated low-FODMAP.

Garlic and onions also contain fructans and are high-FODMAP, as are certain vegetables.
- Galactans may occur in large quantities in a wide range of vegetables, including asparagus, Brussels sprouts, cauliflower, leeks, and mushrooms. Vegetables are an essential part of all diets, and on the full FODMAP list you will find "safe veggies" that are low-FODMAP, including carrots, kale, tomatoes, eggplant, zucchini, and spinach. Legumes are also high in galactans, which is why they are hard to digest. These include various types of beans (baked, pinto, kidney, black, black-eye), chickpeas, split peas, and lentils.
- Polyols, as described above, are sugar alcohols, and include sorbitol, xylitol, maltitol, and mannitol that are added to sugar-free foods and beverages. They are in some vegetables and fruits, and are often added to synthetic sweeteners. Sweeteners that occur naturally and are high in polyols include corn syrup, honey, and agave syrup. But ordinary table sugar and maple syrup are low-FODMAP.

Benefits of the FODMAP Diet

Given the range of disruptive and debilitating symptoms that are triggered by high-FODMAP foods in sensitive individuals, when these symptoms are reduced or eliminated, the benefits are significant. Conditions that were previously unresponsive to medications and other treatments are relieved, and on a natural basis, without drugs or medicines. Digestive disturbances are brought under control or gone, immune system responses like inflammation, and their effects, are diminished, and the previously affected person can enjoy an appreciably improved quality of life.

Low FODMAPs Foods and Your Health

As you now are aware, the range of disease-caused digestive disorders extends to irritable bowel syndrome (IBS), irritable bowel disease (IBD, including Crohn's disease and ulcerative colitis), and leaky gut syndrome, so it may be difficult to determine the precise cause. The low-FODMAP diet has been tested and studied principally among patients suffering from IBS, but the effects are believed to have similar results in treating IBD and leaky gut. The goal is to bring symptoms like stomach pain and cramps, gas and bloating, and diarrhea or constipation, to an end.

It is estimated that most of the 14% of Americans with IBS are not aware that it is the cause of their symptoms; they know they have a serious problem, but they don't know what it is. They become dependent on prescribed medications, or more often, on an assortment of OTC pain relievers, gas, bloating and diarrhea treatments, and acid reflux and indigestion relievers. This is not to diminish the importance of medicines prescribed by physicians, but the optimal solution is to eliminate the causes of the diseases, rather than simply to temporarily reduce the symptoms.

Reduced Digestive Symptoms

The goal of the FODMAP diet is very focused: it is not to lose weight, build muscle mass, or to prevent cardiovascular disease, as important as it is to protect your cardiovascular health. The goal of the three phases of the FODMAP diet is to reduce, or if possible, to eliminate the symptoms of digestive disorders, whether from IBS, IBD, leaky gut, or any undiagnosed disease or condition.

This is especially relevant to IBS, which has no definitive cause, but is known to be responsive to dietary changes: A Monash University study in 2011 found that that a low-FODMAP diet helped 76% of IBS patients, who reported reduction of symptoms, and a resultant upswing in their quality of life.

While the research is less conclusive for other digestive disorders, a low-FODMAP diet is proving effective in bringing relief in the majority of cases, including IBD's two most prominent disorders, Crohn's disease and ulcerative colitis, both of which are autoimmune-caused diseases of the digestive system. Crohn's disease may affect any part of the GI tract, while ulcerative colitis generally only affects the colon, or large intestine.

Some gastroenterologists believe that IBD and IBS may be sufficiently similar to be subtypes of the same disease. If this is a reality, then a low-FODMAP diet could improve symptoms in some cases of IBD. As verification, during a study of 72 IBD patients, a little over half of the patients reported symptoms had definitely improved after three months of a low-FODMAP diet.

Patients with IBS and IBD report less gas and bloating, even after meals, reduced incidents of loose bowels and diarrhea, less constipation, and reduced episodes of intense stomach pain and cramps. Further verification of the value of a low-FODMAP diet was reported in a March 2015 meta-analysis of 22 studies of IBD patients, including clinical trials that compared patients who followed the low-FODMAP diet with patients that did not. The analysis, reported by the *National Library of Medicine* (2015), included six randomized clinical trials and 16 non-randomized trials. There was a statistically significant decrease in IBS symptoms overall among the individuals on a low-FODMAP diet. They experienced measurably reduced severity of symptoms of abdominal pain, bloating, distended abdomen, and overall symptoms.

Reduced Inflammation

Among the benefits of the FODMAP diet, one of the most important is the reduction and control of inflammation. Studies at Monash University in Melbourne, where the FODMAP diet was co-developed, have found positive results in reducing the symptoms of IBD, which, you will recall, is *inflammatory* bowel disease, and includes Crohn's disease and ulcerative colitis.

If you have IBD or other digestive disorder, inflammation can cause the lining of the small intestine, and other parts of the GI tract, to become highly sensitive, and susceptible to infection. Further, when the lining of the small intestine is inflamed, nutrients may not be able to pass completely through to the bloodstream, leading to malnutrition and weight loss. Eliminating inflammation will ensure the healing and recovery of these critical digestive processes.

Another possible condition that inflammation can cause is leaky gut, which allows bacteria and toxins to enter the bloodstream. The FODMAP diet is considered to be invaluable in reducing leaky gut syndrome by ending intestinal inflammation.

Reducing chronic inflammation allows the immune system to normalize and stop sending signals to the brain to initiate the defensive sympathetic, fight-or-flight response, which keeps the body running in high gear, and causing a range of autoimmune responses. Bringing down inflammation by inducing the calming parasympathetic response lowers the heart rate, breathing rate, blood pressure levels, and permits the digestive process to resume normally. Additional benefits include reduced stress and anxiety.

Improved Quality of Life

As a consequence of reducing GI tract symptoms through a FODMAP diet, there are psychological benefits, as well. Relieving physical symptoms leads to reduced stress, which not only lowers immune responses like inflammation but helps bring down tendencies towards anxiety and depression. Additional life quality benefits include an increased sense of self-esteem, and an improved body image, increased energy, vibrancy, and vitality, and improved sexual and social functionalities. The FODMAP diet has the potential to help a person recover and feel they have been restored to a long-ago remembered normalcy, with greatly diminished health concerns.

Imagine a person who has been troubled by Crohn's disease or IBS for years, with little or no relief despite seeing specialists, trying different medications, and even experimenting with alternative medicines and even acupuncture. This person's quality of life has been continuously disrupted by bouts of gastric pain, embarrassing gas and bloating, as well as other symptoms. Then, within a couple of weeks, things start to change.

During the elimination phase of the low-FODMAP diet, the foods that have been causing the disorder have been removed, and with their removal, the symptoms of the disorder begin to diminish and then disappear. It seems like a miracle, but it's nothing more than a simple cause and effect reaction. The source (or sources) of the gastric distress has been removed. The pain and cramps are over, there is no more making excuses running to the toilet; no need to say "No" to invitations. Normalcy has returned.

Gradually, the microbiome's population of beneficial bacteria recover, and the person's entire digestive system achieves balance or equilibrium. This will take some time, so in the second and third phases of the FODMAP diet it is very important to be careful to reintroduce foods individually, and to be alert to any recurring digestive symptoms. That's the warning that a food that triggers sensitivity has come back into the diet, and needs to be removed permanently.

Limitations and Concerns

Unlike most other diets, the FODMAP diet is very strict and limiting, especially in its initial elimination phase (which will be explained in the following chapters). In effect, you are eliminating, albeit temporarily, a very broad range of foods, including many which are considered essential for nutrition. It becomes necessary to be attentive to what is being eliminated and be sure to compensate with complementary foods that are low-FODMAP. Here are some of the key concerns, and recommended solutions.

It isn't always easy. A person who is enthusiastic about trying the FODMAP diet may find it hard to stop eating many, or even most, of the foods they are accustomed to. The elimination phase may be as short as two weeks before foods are gradually reintroduced, but that can be a slow process since the foods need to be brought back into the diet individually. The key is to be well informed about how to substitute low-FODMAP foods for high-FODMAP foods and to have the patience to get through the early, most restrictive days.

Following the diet can be challenging when eating in restaurants, when taking out foods, or when dining in someone's home. It's one thing to be on a salt-free diet, or requesting reduced portion sizes; it's another to not be able to eat many vegetables, fruits, grains, and beans, or dairy products. It may be best to forgo eating out or taking out meals during the early phase of the low-FODMAP diet.

It's restrictive. Nutritionists do not recommend following the FODMAP diet long-term because of its very restrictive nature. Some may worry that followers of the diet may not be able to meet many of their nutritional requirements. For this reason, some experts advocate that those who follow a low-FODMAP diet be under the supervision or guidance of a competent dietician, nutritionist, or other health professional. The alternative is to be fully informed of how to balance your diet nutritionally, especially during the restrictive elimination phase.

For vegetarians and vegans and others on already restricted diets, like those with food allergies, or who follow religiously dictated diets, need to take precautions to maintain good nutrition on the low-FODMAP diet. It can be difficult for them, when additional dietary restrictions are added, to meet their nutritional needs and eat a variety of low-FODMAP foods. Vegans and vegetarians, and others who avoid eating animal products are counseled to get their protein from low-FODMAP sources, including nuts and seeds, soybeans (sold as edamame) and other soy products like tofu, and from alternative grains and cereals like wholegrain quinoa, tempeh, oats, buckwheat, and amaranth.

Since digestive issues are common during pregnancy, especially constipation, there may be a temptation to use a low-FODMAP diet to regain regularity. But there are no conclusive studies to validate the safety of this restrictive diet, and given the high importance of good, complete nutrition, a low-FODMAP diet is not recommended. Pregnant women should reduce constipation and other digestive disorders with medications approved by their doctors. Similarly, there are no studies to support a low-FODMAP diet for children.

To avoid nutritional deficiencies, those following a restrictive low-FODMAP diet may have to replace basic foods with more costly alternatives like certain types of imported fruits and safe to eat cereals, like using buckwheat, amaranth, and quinoa, instead of wheat. These incremental costs are not covered by medical insurance and could result in skewing FODMAP diets to higher income patients.

Healthy intestinal flora requires nutritious food in the intestines to feed upon and to thrive and survive. Some species of beneficial bacteria, including Bifidobacteria, tend to prefer foods that are high-FODMAPs. If confined to a low-FODMAP diet, these bacterial populations may decrease. You need these good bacteria to ferment short-chain carbohydrate molecules in the intestine and produce short-chain fatty acids

(SCFAs) like butyrate, which nourish cells lining the large intestine. Therefore, some high-FODMAP food may be needed to ensure optimal intestinal health. If you are not challenged by IBS or IBD, a low-FODMAP diet may be harmful to your gut microbiome. This is why it's important to check with a doctor before starting the FODMAP diet.

Now, let's move on to the FODMAP diet itself, and learn about low, medium, and high-FODMAP foods.

Chapter 6:

FODMAP Diet Chart

At this point in our study of the gastrointestinal system, you know that certain types of food can trigger a number of digestive issues. Specifically, foods categorized as FODMAPs, which are high in fermentable carbohydrates, can cause digestive system symptoms, including gas and bloating, diarrhea or constipation, cramps, and other debilitating stomach pain. FODMAPs are classified as either high or low in their sensitivity-inducing short-chain carbohydrates and sugar alcohols.

By identifying, and then restricting high-FODMAP foods from your digestive system, you can experience almost immediate relief of GI tract symptoms, especially in cases of irritable bowel syndrome (IBS).

Rating the FODMAPs

This chapter will provide their lists of foods by category and will identify if they are high or low in FODMAPs. Additional, up-to-date lists are also provided, so you will be able to follow the FODMAP diet with clear identification of what must go, at least temporarily, and what can stay.

The origins of the FODMAP are a team of researchers at Monash University's Department of Gastroenterology from Melbourne, Australia, identified certain short-chain carbohydrates in food that for some people, may be indigestible and poorly absorbed in the small intestine; instead they are consumed by certain microbe in the large intestine, creating digestive system disorders. The team came up with the acronym FODMAPs for these fermentable carbohydrates and sugar alcohols.

Subsequently, Monash University and King's College, London, joined forces and collaborated in developing the concept of FODMAPs, and food lists that separate foods by their saccharide content. The team measured the FODMAP content of hundreds of different foods in categories that include vegetables, fruit, cereals and grains, nuts and seeds, legumes, processed food, and dairy products. Their analysis enabled the researchers to develop the low-FODMAP diet. They subsequently applied this low-FODMAP diet in clinical studies and confirmed that low FODMAPs diet can reduce the symptoms of Irritable Bowel Syndrome (IBS) and other digestive diseases, which we now know includes IBD's Crohn's disease and ulcerative colitis.

Their published findings of saccharide levels suggest that high-FODMAP foods contain more than one of the following fermentable, short-chain carbohydrates and sugar alcohols:

- Monosaccharides: 0.2 grams more fructose than glucose, as found in certain fruits and vegetables.
- Disaccharides: 4.0 grams of lactose, typically found in milk and other dairy products.
- Oligosaccharides: 0.3 grams of fructans or galactooligosaccharides, often found in grains and some vegetables.
- Polyols: 0.3 grams of sorbitol or mannitol, found in sweeteners.

The lists will present you with foods you may safely continue in your diet because they are low-FODMAPs, but keep in mind that you cannot make determinations about high-FODMAPs simply by reviewing the lists, and deciding what to stop eating. You must follow the three phases of the FODMAP diet, as detailed in the next chapter. That is the only way to accurately identify the carbohydrates that you are sensitive to and remove them from your diet.

The Perspective

We can't guess which foods are high-FODMAP, and which are low-FODMAP. It is only due to the extensive analyses by the research team that patiently tested each food to determine whether it contains important quantities of monosaccharides, disaccharides, and oligosaccharides, the short-chain carbohydrates and sugar alcohols that can trigger IBS, IBD, and other GI tract symptoms and disturbances.

Before we plunge into the long lists of high and low-FODMAP foods, we need to appreciate that many foods and beverages must be eliminated initially on a low-FODMAP diet, and these include certain fruits and vegetables, legumes, including lentils and beans, popular grains like wheat and rye, dairy products that contain lactose, and sweeteners including honey, high fructose corn syrup, and sweetening additives.

On the other hand, a wide range of foods are low-FODMAP and may continue to be safely enjoyed without hesitation (within reasonable caloric limits, of course). Just as certain fruits and vegetables are high-FODMAPs, others are rated low. Lactose-free dairy is okay, as are grains like rice, oats, and quinoa, and soybeans, moderate amounts of nuts and seeds, plus eggs, unprocessed meat and fish (which are primarily protein and fat, with minimal carbohydrates). There are curious exceptions:

- Gin, vodka, and whisky are low-FODMAP, but rum, alone among all alcoholic beverages, is high-FODMAP. Why? The other beverages are distilled from grain, which is mostly high-FODMAP, while rum is distilled from sugar, which is low-FODMAP. The answer for the grain-based spirits may be that the fermentation process of turning sugars and starches into alcohol, also converts the FODMAPs into more complex molecules that are less appealing to the

- bad bacteria in the colon. But why the sugarcane used in making rum doesn't convert the saccharides remains a mystery.
- Another example of the effects of fermentation is ordinary bread made with wheat and rye is high-FODMAP, but sourdough bread is low, even when made with wheat or rye. There is a logical cause and effect: the fermentation process of lactobacillus bacteria, which creates the "sour" in sourdough, reduces the FODMAPs as the dough is going through its many hours of rising and curing.

It is important to underscore that the FODMAP diet is not for everyone. Unlike popular diets, like the Mediterranean and keto diets, which offer extensive health benefits, including weight management, and preventing obesity, diabetes, and heart disease, the FODMAP diet is specifically for people who are experiencing IBS, IBD (including Crohn's disease and ulcerative colitis). In this context, the FODMAP diet can stop the symptoms of these digestive system diseases, and lead the person back gradually in the second and third phases to a diet that is much less restrictive than the first, exclusion phase. A person who has no digestive disorder symptoms will not experience changes or improvements after several weeks of following the exclusion phase.

FODMAPs By Food Category

As a reminder, all high-FODMAPs that are in a person's diet are to be eliminated in phase 1, while low-FODMAPs may be consumed during all phases of the FODMAP diet. For the diet to be effective in identifying the foods that are the causes of the symptoms, there can be no exceptions about not eating any high-FODMAP foods during phase 1; elimination means elimination. Given that the elimination phase can be as short as two or three weeks, it is not an unreasonable expectation to surrender the high-FODMAP foods, especially since a wide range of safe substitutes is available from the long list of low-FODMAPs:

- So while you might miss apples, peaches, and cherries for a while, you are safe to eat melons, grapes, oranges, and strawberries instead.
- Similarly, you'll be giving up asparagus, green peas, mushrooms, and onions but will be free to enjoy green beans, eggplant, broccoli, cucumbers, and zucchini.
- If you love drinking cow's milk, you can continue to do so during the elimination phase by switching to lactose-free milk or any of the many alternatives, like almond milk and soy protein milk.
- Most meat sources of protein are safe to continue, as long as they're not marinated or preserved.

- Bread, cereals, and pasta made with wheat or rye will not be available to you, but many other grains, like rice, quinoa, and buckwheat can fill in with added benefits of rich flavor and high protein and fiber. And sourdough bread, as we've mentioned, is an okay low-FODMAP food.

The first list is brief, published by Monash University on their website and accessible online. The university also has an app to download; other apps are also available and provide lists of high and low-FODMAP foods by category. The second, more extensive list follows the Monash list.

Monash University Sample FODMAP Diet Food List

Food Category	High FODMAP Foods	Low FODMAP Alternatives
Fruits	Apples, Canned Fruit, Cherries, Dried Fruits, Mangos, Nectarines and Peaches, Pears, Plums, and Watermelons.	Cantaloupes and Honeydews, Grapes, Kiwis, Mandarins and Oranges, Pineapples, and Strawberries.
Vegetables	Asparagus, Artichokes, Cauliflower, Garlic,	Aubergine (Eggplant), Bell Peppers, Bok Choy, Broccoli, Carrots,

	Green Peas, Leeks, Mushrooms, Onions, Scallions, and Sugar Snap Peas.	Celery, Cucumbers, Green Beans, Lettuce, Okra, Olives, Potatoes, Rhubarb, Spinach, Sweet Potatoes, Tomatoes, Yellow Squash, and Zucchini.
Dairy and Substitutes	Cow's Milk and Cream, Cream Cheese, Goat's Milk, Sheep's Milk, Custards, Evaporated Milk, Ice Cream and Gelato, Soy Milk (made from whole Soybeans), and Yogurt.	Milk Beverages made from Almonds, Oats, and Soy Protein, Lactose-Free Milk, Soft Cheeses like Brie, Camembert, Cottage Cheese, Feta, and Hard Cheeses like Cheddar, Parmesan, and Swiss.
Protein Sources	Most Dried Legumes (Beans, Chickpeas, Lentils, Split Peas), Marinated Beef, Poultry, Seafood (fresh, frozen, canned), and Processed Meats, including Bacon, Salami, Sausages.	Eggs, plain Beef, Poultry, Lamb, Pork, Fish and other Seafood (fresh, frozen, canned), Tempeh and Tofu (firm, from Soy). Also canned, and rinsed Chickpeas, and Lentils.
Bread, Grains, and Cereals	Wheat-based Bread, Biscuits, Cereals, Pasta, Snacks, or made with Rye, Spelt, and Barley.	Buckwheat, Corn, Millet, Quinoa, and Rice-based Bread, Cereals, Snacks, Pasta, and Sourdough Bread.
Sugars, Sweeteners,	Agave, Honey, High-Fructose Corn Syrup,	Dark Chocolate, Maple Syrup, Rice Malt Syrup,

and Confections	Milk Chocolate, Sugar-Free Confectioneries and Sweeteners, and Additives, including Xylitol, Sorbitol, and Maltitol.	Sugar, Sucralose (Splenda), and Stevia.
Nuts and Seeds	Cashews and Pistachios	Almonds, Hazelnuts, Macadamias, Peanuts, Pecans, Pine Nuts, Walnuts, Chia, Flax, Pumpkin, Sesame, and Sunflower Seeds.
Snacks	Made with Wheat, and Rye, or with Garlic or Onions.	Corn Chips, Potato Chips, Popcorn, Rice Crackers.
Condiments	Agave, Curry, or Quince paste, Caviar Dip, Hummus, Pesto sauce, Relish, Sauces with Garlic or Onions, and Stock Cubes.	Salt and Pepper, and most Dried Herbs, Sauces without Onions or Garlic, Ketchup, Mayonnaise, Mustard, Oils, Soy Sauce, Vinegar (Balsamic, Cider, Malt, Red Wine), Worcester Sauce.
Beverages	Apple Juice and Cider, Coconut Water, some Herbal Teas (Chamomile, Fennel, Oolong). Rum, Dessert Wines, Mixed Cocktails.	Black and Green Teas, Coffee, Fresh Orange, Lemon, and Lime Juice, and Tomato Juice. Red and White Wines, Beer, Gin, Vodka, Whisky, Water.

Source: *Monash University*, High and Low FODMAP Foods (2019).

FODMAP Diet: Full List by Food Groups

Since Monash University published its list of high and low-FODMAP foods, other organizations have reviewed the studies and published their own lists. Among the many available for review, the *Diet vs. Disease* (2019) list is extensive and easy to use, with a large range of foods organized by category and listed individually. In addition to the high and low ratings, in some cases foods are rated as medium FODMAP, meaning they are okay in small quantities and low frequency of consumption.

FODMAP Vegetables

High FODMAP To Be Avoided	Medium FODMAP Enjoy Sparingly	Low FODMAP Enjoy Completely
Asparagus Artichoke Cauliflower	Beetroot (½ cup) Brussels sprouts (4 small)	Alfalfa Arugula (Rocket) Asian & collard

Garlic	Butternut squash (½ cup)	greens
Leek (white part)		Bean sprouts
Mushrooms (Button, Portobello, Shiitake)	Corn (½ cob)	Bell peppers (Capsicum)
	Olives (Green or Black)	Broccoli
		Cabbage
	Snow peas (5 pods)	Carrots
Onions		Celery
Peas	Spaghetti squash (1 cup)	Celery root (Celeriac)
Scallions (white part)		
	Sweet potato (½)	Chard (Silverbeet)
		Chili (red or green)
		Cucumbers
		Edamame
		Eggplant (Aubergine)
		Endive
		Fennel (bulb and leaves)

		Ginger and Galangal
		Green beans
		Kale
		Lettuce (all types)
		Mushrooms (canned, Oyster, Shimeji)
		Okra
		Potato
		Pumpkin/Squash (Japanese)
		Radish
		Rhubarb
		Scallion (green parts only)
		Seaweed/Nori
		Spinach (baby or English)
		Tomatoes

		Turnip
		Rutabaga
		Water chestnut
		Yam
		Zucchini (courgette)

Source: *Diet vs. Disease*. Low FODMAP Food List: What Can You Eat On a Low FODMAP Diet? (2019).

FODMAP Fruits

High FODMAP To Be Avoided	Medium FODMAP Enjoy Sparingly	Low FODMAP Enjoy Completely
Apples	Avocado	Blueberries
Apricots	Bananas (firm/green, medium-size)	Grapes
Ripe bananas		Lemons
Blackberries		Limes
Cherries	Cantaloupe (½ cup)	Mandarins
Grapefruit	Coconut (desiccated, ½	Oranges
Mango		Passion fruit

	cup)	Raspberries
Nectarines	Honeydew melon (½ cup)	Strawberries
Peaches		
Pears	Kiwi fruit (2 small)	
Plums		
Raisins, Sultanas	Pineapple (1 cup)	
Watermelon		

Source: *Diet vs. Disease.* Low FODMAP Food List: What Can You Eat On a Low FODMAP Diet? (2019).

FODMAP Proteins

High FODMAP To Be Avoided	Medium FODMAP Enjoy Sparingly	Low FODMAP Enjoy Completely
Baked beans	Bacon (pure, minimally processed)	Beef
Black beans		Chicken
Canned meats		Lamb
Cannellini beans	Chickpeas (canned, rinsed)	Pork (including unprocessed ham)
Chickpeas (dried)		
Cold cuts		Turkey

Lentils (dried)		Fish, Seafood (fresh, canned, smoked)
Marinated meats		
Mixed beans		Eggs
Processed meat		Lentils (canned, rinsed)
Salami, sausage		
Tofu (silken)		Lima, mung beans
Soybeans		Quorn
		Tempeh
		Tofu (firm)

Source: *Diet vs. Disease*. Low FODMAP Food List: What Can You Eat On a Low FODMAP Diet? (2019).

FODMAPs Grains

High FODMAP To Be Avoided	Medium FODMAP Enjoy Sparingly	Low FODMAP Enjoy Completely
Barley	Cacao powder (2 teaspoons)	Amaranth
Besan flour		Arrowroot
Cereal, muesli, granola with	Oats, Oatmeal, Oat flour	Buckwheat flour
		Cereal (no wheat,

wheat, honey, or dried fruit Chickpea flour Coconut flour Rye flour Soy flour Spelt flour Wheat flour All foods made with high FODMAP flour (cakes, cookies, biscuits, bread, muffins)		honey, or dried fruit) Corn flakes Corn/Maize flour Corn tortillas Muesli (no fruit) Rice Krispies Sourdough bread (no yeast) Spirulina Tapioca flour Teff

Source: *Diet vs. Disease.* Low FODMAP Food List: What Can You Eat On a Low FODMAP Diet? (2019).

FODMAP Condiments, Dips, Sweets, Sweeteners, and Spreads

High FODMAP To Be Avoided	Medium FODMAP Enjoy Sparingly	Low FODMAP Enjoy Completely
Agave	None	BBQ sauce

Chips or snacks with onion or garlic powder		Chocolate (dark, 85% cacao or more is ideal)
Curry paste		
Dried fruit		Corn chips
Gravy mix		Cookies or biscuits made with low FODMAP flours
High fructose corn syrup		
		Jello
Honey		Ketchup/Tomato sauce
Hummus		
Inulin		Golden syrup
Isomalt		Maple syrup
		Margarine
Jam (real strawberry jam and marmalade okay)		Mayonnaise
Maltitol		Mint sauce
Mannitol		Mint jelly
Milk and white chocolate		Miso paste
		Mustard
Pasta sauces		Peanut butter
Sorbitol		Potato chips (plain,

Tzatziki		salted)
Xylitol		Popcorn
		Rice crackers, rice cakes crispbread
		Sweeteners (Equal, Stevia, and Splenda)
		Shrimp paste
		Soy, fish, and oyster sauce
		Sweet and sour sauce
		Vanilla essence
		Vegemite/Marmite
		Vinegar (balsamic, malt, red wine)
		Worcestershire sauce

Source: *Diet vs. Disease.* Low FODMAP Food List: What Can You Eat On a Low FODMAP Diet? (2019).

FODMAP Nuts and Seeds

High FODMAP To Be Avoided	Medium FODMAP Enjoy Sparingly	Low FODMAP Enjoy Completely
Cashews	None	Almonds
Pistachios		Brazil nuts
		Chia seeds
		Flaxseeds
		Hazelnuts
		Macadamia nuts
		Peanut butter and almond butter
		Peanuts
		Pecans
		Pine nuts
		Pumpkin seeds
		Sesame seeds
		Sunflower seeds
		Walnuts

Source: *Diet vs. Disease.* Low FODMAP Food List: What Can You Eat On a Low FODMAP Diet? (2019)

FODMAP Dairy and Dairy Substitutes

High FODMAP To Be Avoided	Medium FODMAP Enjoy Sparingly	Low FODMAP Enjoy Completely
Cow's milk, cream Cream cheese Goat's milk Oat milk Sheep's milk Soy milk (made from soybeans)	Canned coconut milk	Butter Cheese (all firm varieties) Cottage cheese Ricotta cheese Lactose-free milk Lactose-free yogurt (plain) Milk, nondairy: almond, hemp, quinoa, rice soy (made from soy protein)

Source: *Diet vs. Disease.* Low FODMAP Food List: What Can You Eat On a Low FODMAP Diet? (2019).

FODMAP Beverages and Drinks

High FODMAP To Be Avoided	Medium FODMAP Enjoy Sparingly	Low FODMAP Enjoy Completely
Apple cider	None	Black tea, green tea
Apple juice		Chocolate (drinking, cacao-based, not carob)
Coconut water		
Herbal tea varieties (Chamomile, Fennel, Oolong)		Coffee (no milk)
		Cranberry juice
Mango juice		Dandelion tea
Pear cider		Fresh orange juice
Pear juice		Lemon juice
Sodas with high fructose corn syrup		Lime juice
		Peppermint tea
Cocktails		Tomato juice
Rum		Water
		Beer (gluten-free)
		Champagne

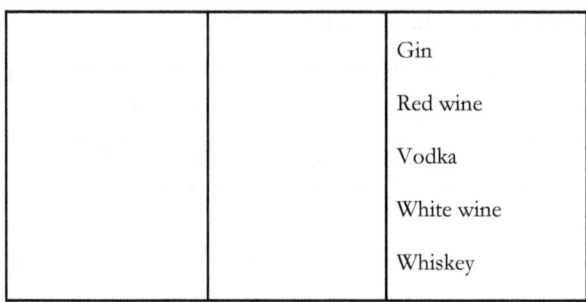

Source: *Diet vs. Disease.* Low FODMAP Food List: What Can You Eat On a Low FODMAP Diet? (2019).

You have seen that high-FODMAPs are in a broad assortment of foods, including vegetables and fruits, cereals and grains, seeds and nuts, legumes, including beans and lentils, dairy foods, and some beverages. The only category mostly free of high-FODMAPs includes high protein meat and fish. Following the FODMAP diet can be challenging because you always have to pay attention, you cannot just guess which foods will be high-FODMAPs or low-FODMAPs.

By gaining a fundamental understanding about the foods that contain FODMAPs, and to what degree, will make following the three-step FODMAP diet easier long term and helps you to avoid the unwanted and unpleasant symptoms of IBS, or IBD's Crohn's disease and ulcerative colitis.

Summary of FODMAPs By Food Group

While the lists will be your standard, go-to resource to determine the FODMAP status of almost every food you might consider here is a summary of the types of FODMAP saccharides in each of the food groups.

Vegetables: The principal FODMAPs found in many vegetables are fructans and mannitol, with fructans being particularly rich in artichokes, garlic, and onions, leeks and scallions, or spring onions. Cauliflower, mushrooms, and snow peas are particularly rich in mannitol.

Fruit: The FODMAPs present abundantly in fruit are sorbitol and excess fructose (fruit sugar), especially in apples, cherries, figs, mangoes, pears, watermelon, and dried fruit. Fruits that are rich in sorbitol are apples, blackberries, as well as peaches, and plums. As is evident some fruits contain both fructose and sorbitol: apples, cherries, and pears.

Proteins: Meat, poultry, and fish are very high in protein, they are low in carbohydrates and all FODMAPs, and are safe to include in a low-FODMAP diet. However, if they are marinated or served with sauces containing onions or garlic, or are heavily processed, like canned meats, sausages, or salami, they become high-FODMAP. Eggs are also high in protein and low in FODMAPs. The principal FODMAP to be found in legumes and pulses is GOS, with the greatest amount in beans, especially red kidney beans, plus split-peas, falafels, and baked beans of many varieties.

Grains: Fructans are the principal FODMAPs found in cereals and grains, with smaller amounts of GOS (galactooligosaccharides) present. The foods especially rich in fructans include wholegrain wheat and rye bread, and breakfast cereals and muesli that contain wheat, plus wheat-based pasta and rye crispbread.

Sugars and sweeteners: Foods and beverages that are sweetened with sugar usually contain fructose and sugar polyols (erythritol, sorbitol, xylitol). Check the food labels to identify high-FODMAP sugars, particularly in beverages and confectionery that are artificially sweetened. Ingredients that are high in FODMAP sugar include high fructose corn syrup and honey. Products and ingredients that are advertised as sugar-free may be high-FODMAPs. Dark chocolate, table or granulated sugar, maple syrup, and rice malt syrup are low-FODMAPs.

Condiments and spices: Since some condiments, dips, marinades, and sauces contain onion and garlic, they are high-FODMAP. Low-FODMAP choices include BBQ sauce, chutney, cranberry sauce, mayonnaise, and soy sauce.

Nuts and seeds: Chia, flax, pumpkin, sunflower, and most other seeds are low-FODMAP. A few nuts—cashews and pistachios—contain GOS and fructans and are high-FODMAPs. Most other nuts are low-FODMAP, including almonds, hazelnuts, macadamias, peanuts, pecans, pine nuts, and walnuts.

Dairy and dairy substitutes: Lactose, or milk sugar, is the FODMAP found in dairy products, notably milk, soft cheeses, like cream and cottage cheeses, and yogurt. But many dairy foods are naturally low in their lactose content, including butter and an array of hard cheeses. So dairy is not automatically excluded from a low-FODMAP diet, and lactose-free milk and yogurt are low-FODMAP. Dairy substitutes like almond and soy protein milk are low-FODMAP, as well.

Beverages: Since many beverages contain fruit extracts or sugar substitutes, they may be high in the same saccharides: excess fructose (fruit sugar), or sugar polyols (erythritol, sorbitol, xylitol), or combinations.

As you review the lists, try to become familiar with the foods that you like, but are high-FODMAPs and will need to be eliminated. How to do that is explained in the next chapter.

Chapter 7:

Three Phases of the FODMAP Diet

The generally recommended and prescribed FODMAP diet is broken down into three stages: elimination, gradual identification of sensitivities, and personalization, which results in a long-term, or continuing diet plan that eliminates only specific foods that cause problems. What at first appears to be a formidable challenge, with hundreds of foods to be concerned about, is actually quite manageable when you see the most difficult phase is short. You will not have to give up all the foods you love and are accustomed to; rather, you will be isolating and identifying what may be a limited number of foods that are the source of your digestive issues.

To underscore this point, do not imagine that you will be on a low-FODMAP diet forever. Most people, even those with IBS and IBD, are not sensitive to all high-FODMAP foods. Once individual high-FODMAP foods have been cleared, they may be returned to your diet and enjoyed without concern.

Overview of the Three Phases

Before getting into the details of how to manage the three phases of the FODMAP diet, this overview will give you a perspective of what each phase involves. Always keep in mind that the FODMAP diet is not a steady or continuous diet, such as the Mediterranean diet, which is meant to be a life-long discipline. The FODMAP diet, in contrast, is evolutionary and meant to refine your diet and let you continue to enjoy as many of your favorite foods as possible. Within a matter of months, you can be eating both low and high-FODMAP foods with confidence, once you have eliminated the sensitivities.

The first phase is the most challenging, because it removes a wide range of popular foods from the diet, albeit, temporarily. This elimination phase is also known as the restriction phase. During this phase, all foods rated high in FODMAPs are removed from the diet for a period lasting from two to six weeks.

If a person's digestive tract is sensitive to any high-FODMAP foods, and if all high-FODMAP foods are removed from the diet, then the digestive symptoms should disappear during the elimination phase. This confirms that the IBD or IBS or other intestinal disorder is definitely caused by certain carbohydrates in the diet.

This phase is usually the most difficult step of the FODMAP process because so many foods that people like contain potentially risky carbohydrates, and all high-FODMAPs must be eliminated, at least initially. Researchers who developed the FODMAP diet caution that information has evolved, and earlier versions of the diet may not be up to date, so be sure to refer to the categories of FODMAPs in the previous chapter, which are based on the latest findings.

The second phase enables the reintroduction of high-FODMAP foods by identifying sensitivities: after the high-FODMAPs have been eliminated or importantly reduced from the diet, nutritionists recommend a process of carefully testing high-FODMAP food groups individually, i.e., reintroducing one at a time. This disciplined approach allows you to test your response to each food group.

Different people respond differently to carbohydrates. You might be highly sensitive to fructans and not be able to tolerate wheat, rye, and barley, while another person is okay with fructans, but can't handle lactose, the disaccharide in milk and other daily products. This underscore testing carbohydrates individually to ensure the exact "culprits" are identified. Each high-FODMAP food that is returned to the diet and tested should be experienced for three days or more, to give it a chance to reveal its acceptability and safety, or to see if it provokes a digestive system reaction.

For example, if you want to test if you can resume eating honey, which is high in fructose monosaccharides, you might have one teaspoon a day for three or four days. If no digestive symptoms return, honey can return safely to your diet. But if symptoms return during the honey trial, you will know that it should not return to your diet.

Upon completion of the testing phase, when you know which food groups you can tolerate, and which food groups you cannot tolerate, and which provoke symptoms, you can begin to reintroduce the tolerable foods into your daily, ongoing diet. Your goal is to return to eating as many FODMAPs as you safely can, to reduce the risks of nutritional deficiencies, and to avoid depriving good bacteria in the intestines of the foods they thrive on.

Given that some of us may have unique sensitivities that are caused by specific FODMAP foods, it is important not to assume that we need to complete the personalization phase to make sure we are getting optimal nutrition, without provoking our digestive systems. In other words, many foods will resume their place in your diet during phase 2. But be aware that over time our body can change, and some high-FODMAP foods that are found to aggravate your GI tract today, may be retested in a few months to see if your body has developed tolerance.

Phase 1: Elimination

The first phase of the FODMAP diet is the elimination of all high-FODMAP foods, which includes every food listed in the high-FODMAPs columns in the previous chapter. For this phase to be successful, there can be no exceptions, no matter how tempting. In most instances, sensitivity can be triggered by even a trace of a food that contains an oligosaccharide, or another type of short-chain saccharide, that your gut is sensitive to. Fortunately, while you may find it tough to accomplish a total elimination of many foods you like and are accustomed to, the elimination phase does not have to be endured for long; for good reasons, it should be relatively short.

The Need for a Brief Elimination Phase

The elimination phase is very important, yet it is relatively brief because it does not take long to bring digestive disorder symptoms to an end when all high-FODMAP foods are removed from the diet. And it is important to return many essential foods and nutrients to the diet sooner, rather than later to protect your health.

For example, the elimination phase deprives you of essential sources of fiber that you normally obtain from vegetables, fruits, and whole grains. As a consequence of an extended absence of fiber, you could experience constipation, aggravating what might already be a problem, or constipation if it wasn't already an IBS or IBD symptom you experienced.

You also need fiber to maintain good health. Cardiologists warn that a low level of fiber in the diet is associated with elevated cholesterol, leading to a higher risk of cardiovascular disease, type 2 diabetes, and possibly colorectal cancer. Fiber also helps with weight control since it suppresses appetite by giving you a sense of fullness or satiety while contributing fewer calories. Dietary fiber helps regulate blood sugar levels, leads to improved digestive system health overall, and enhances the functioning of the immune system.

Fiber and other FODMAP foods are prebiotics, serving as a source of fuel to provide energy for the bacteria in our gut microbiome. Depriving the gut bacteria of nutrients limits their viability and survival, and without them, we can diminish our overall health status while reducing our ability to digest certain foods. In the absence of the usual prebiotic foods, the desperate microbes may turn to the mucus cells that coat the stomach and intestinal linings. As a result, the epithelial cells that form a barrier are thinned, resulting in inflammation of the digestive tract. In some cases, the bacteria may migrate to other parts of the body, triggering immune responses and inflammation.

The rationale for a brief elimination phase is not limited to fiber and other prebiotics. Removing certain food groups for a long time may leave a person susceptible to dietary nutritional deficiencies, including iron, folate, and vitamin B12, which are frequently sourced from whole grains and fortified cereals. Many vegetables and fruits are frequently high in FODMAPs and need to be excluded during the elimination phase. Yet these foods are high in many essential antioxidants, vitamins A, B, and C, and minerals, including iron, calcium, potassium, and zinc.

Taking dairy products out of the diet can cause a reduced intake of vitamin D, calcium, and other nutrients, as well as depriving you of a good source of protein. In aggregate, these deficiencies can result in greater health risks, like anemia, osteoporosis and bone loss, slower healing, and electrolyte imbalances.

Implementing the Elimination Phase

In principle, conducting the elimination phase could not be more simple:

- Review all the lists of high-FODMAP foods and beverages in the previous chapter, and on the day you want to begin the diet, remove all of these potentially sensitivity-activating foods from your diet.
- Follow the Monash University protocol of eating no foods—none!—on the high-FODMAPs list, and selecting only sparingly from the middle column of medium-FODMAP foods. Make the food category low-FODMAP lists your roadmap, and consider the vertical lines of the lists as guardrails to keep you from drifting into the wrong lanes.

Of course, there's a bit more to do for this to go smoothly and work effectively. The following tips and recommendations should be helpful.

Change Your Mindset

Much of the success of a disciplined dietary program begins in the mindset, where self-discipline, thinking, and planning need to be marshaled to get you going and keep you on track.

Resolve that all high-FODMAP foods and beverages will be eliminated; no exceptions, and plan to stop eating out, or socially, if you can, for at least two weeks. If it can't be avoided, plan ahead by checking the menu in advance, so you can leisurely find low-FODMAP food to select, or alert your social host or hostess of your limitations. It's more courteous, and it will let your host do some custom preparation,

Identify the foods on the low-FODMAP lists that you can substitute for the high-FODMAP foods you are most accustomed to eating and drinking.

- For example, as you give up wheat-based bread, cereals, and pasta, be receptive to the idea of switching to the same products, but made instead with amaranth, rice, buckwheat, or quinoa, as alternatives.
- You can easily switch from regular milk and dairy to lactose-free versions; they taste the same and tend to be lower in calories and higher in protein.
- Instead of apples, apricots, and pears, try blueberries, grapes, and strawberries.
- If you prefer a more natural sweetener like honey, which is high-FODMAP, switch over to low-FODMAP pure maple syrup.

Resist temptation to cheat, even just a little, by being tempted to taste any high FODMAP foods. Some food sensitivities can be activated by just a trace of the saccharide molecules that are present in a teaspoon of the food. Keep reminding yourself that this is only for a few weeks, and there's no sense in disrupting the purity of the elimination's identification of what's safe to eat and what's not. Practice positive thinking, and keep telling yourself that you can do this, you've got this.

Behavioral Steps

Getting the job done, by successfully completing the elimination phase, is more than planning, it requires action. These steps will help to get you there.

Make lists and stock up. As you study the lists of FODMAP foods and are learning what you can eat during the elimination phase, it's a practical exercise to start making shopping lists with your new dietary options.

- Normally, you could shop on "autopilot," without thinking too much, because you were shopping for the familiar foods you always have favored. But now, you don't want to be guessing in the market or having to consult this book or other sources of the FODMAP food lists.
- Rather than running out to the market for a few things every day, buying for the week will help prevent you from being out of the right foods, and have only wrong foods available. So plan for a week of all low-FODMAP foods, and put them on your shopping lists (recipes and other ideas are waiting for you in the next chapters).

Go the distance. Don't quit your FODMAP diet prematurely, especially during the elimination phase. Only by staying off all high-FODMAP foods can you determine if your digestive disorder symptoms are caused by high-FODMAP foods, and are not due to a different type of food, or a non-food stimulus. like chronic stress and inflammation, or other immune system reactions.

It generally takes at least two weeks to be sure, but some people find that can eliminate all symptoms within a week. Whether it's two weeks or a bit longer, be patient, and don't resume eating any high-FODMAP foods prematurely. Remind yourself, this phase will be over soon.

Get enough fiber. As noted above, since some of the high-FODMAP foods you will be eliminating during the first phase are a primary source of fiber, if they are not replaced with low-FODMAP foods that are high in fiber, you will risk constipation.

- If you are giving up pistachios, replace them with hazelnuts, almonds, or walnuts. Continue to keep fiber-rich vegetables, from the low-FODMAP list, in your diet; the same with fibrous fruits.
- Give the wheat alternative grains a try, especially the whole grain versions, which are higher in fiber (and other nutrients) than the polished wheat grains used in most bread and pasta. You may need a fiber supplement, like psyllium husk.
- Be aware that if you are not accustomed to a high fiber diet, a sudden introduction of a diet high in insoluble fiber can jolt the intestines,

and cause new digestive stress. Also, be sure to drink enough water to help prevent constipation.

Prepare takeaway meals. It's one thing to follow the low-FODMAP diet at home; it's another when you're out and about, away from your modified kitchen. What to do about lunch and snacks?

Instead of trying your luck at your workplace, school cafeteria, or nearby cafe, keep control of your diet by taking advantage of what you've stocked up on, and toss together low-FODMAP sandwiches, salad bowls, and safe-to-eat chips and other snacks. Allow an extra 10 minutes or so in the morning, so you have time to prep the meals before heading out the door.

Keep a journal. Make a daily note in a log or journal of how you feel, especially as to the symptoms you are experiencing, and if they are diminishing. It will be helpful to you, and to the doctor, dietician, or nutritionist you may be consulting, to know if tangible progress is being made. You can use a scale of one to 10, with one being virtually no abdominal pain, cramps, gas, diarrhea, or other symptoms of IBS, IBD, or other disorder, and 10 being maximum discomfort and disability.

Once you have maintained the elimination phase for at least two weeks, and have been without any symptoms for the last several days, you are ready for the next phase. If the symptoms continue after two weeks, keep the elimination going, up to six weeks, but no longer.

Phase 2: Reintroduction

Transitioning from the elimination phase is predicated on your having successfully eliminated, or appreciably reduced, the symptoms of your digestive tract disease or disorder. Cramps and gas, abdominal pain, chronic diarrhea, or whatever gastrointestinal discomforts and symptoms have been troubling you, have receded, and are being managed by the elimination of all high-FODMAP foods during the previous weeks.

These results confirm that your symptoms are caused by sensitivities to certain foods, and if you continue to avoid the offending high-FODMAP foods, those symptoms should stay away, or at least remain only at much lower levels.

But what if your digestive tract symptoms remain as before, unchanged, and continuing to disrupt your way of life by discomforting and perhaps debilitating you? If you have given the low-FODMAP diet a full opportunity to reduce symptoms, by abstaining without exception from every high-FODMAP food, for up to six weeks without positive results, then you may reasonably conclude that something else is at fault:

- Your IBS, or IBD, or another disease may be caused by chronic stress, and the inflammation and immune responses it causes.
- It may be an imbalance among the bacteria in the intestines, including an invasion of a destructive bacteria strain, like clostridium

difficile, which needs to be treated by insertion of a donor microbiome.
- It is important to report an unsuccessful low-FODMAP diet elimination phase to your doctor, who may want to try further diagnoses or treatments.

The Gradual Introduction of High-FODMAPs

This is the phase that identifies sensitivities to specific high-FODMAP food groups.

Assuming your gut is now relatively calm and at peace with you, it is time to bring back high-FODMAP foods to determine what you can handle and what you cannot. This process should begin promptly to bring essential nutrients back into your diet without delay, and to rebuild the diet of the beneficial bacteria in your intestinal microbiome. These microbes are especially fond of high-FODMAP foods, and they have been deprived of this prebiotic nourishment during the elimination phase

The objective of the FODMAP reintroduction phase is to learn which high-FODMAP foods aggravate your gastrointestinal symptoms, by conducting a sequence of food challenges. This procedure may be described as finding the tolerance level for a high-FODMAP food group. It follows these steps:

At the beginning of each week during this phase of reintroduction, you select one of the high-FODMAP food groups to challenge. You eat a small quantity of one food from that group over three days. On day two, and then on day three, you gradually increase the quantity of the challenge food you will be eating. If you are starting with wheat in the grain group, for example, have a half-slice of wheat bread on day one, a full slice on day two, and one and a half slices on day three. From the fruit group, start with one-third of an apple, then two-thirds, and then an entire apple on day three.

You will monitor your gut symptoms during each challenge to check on your ability to handle or tolerate each FODMAP group.

As you continue this procedure, one food group at a time, you will gradually learn:

- Which high-FODMAP groups cause no sensitivities, and you will be able to enjoy them without restraint.
- Which high-FODMAP food groups you may have to eat less frequently and in smaller quantities.
- Which are the high-FODMAP food groups that cause your symptoms and need to be rarely, if ever, part of your diet if you plan to maintain a calm and symptom-free gastrointestinal system.

You may look forward to joining most people who discover that their level of tolerance is good for most high-FODMAP food groups, and they are able to develop an extensive diet that includes a wide assortment of high and low-FODMAP foods and maintain this diet for many years.

Finding High-FODMAP Trigger Foods

Two types of discoveries are inevitable during the reintroductions phase. Some foods and food groups may be found to be perfectly harmless and be able to return to your diet, and other foods may be found that trigger gastrointestinal disease symptoms. This is to be expected, and should not cause panic. This is a scientific finding, not a setback.

When new symptoms are initiated by a high-FODMAP food, stop eating the food, and allow it to pass through the GI tract; this usually takes two or three days. During this time, no other food challenges should begin. Once the symptoms are gone, it is safe to resume the reintroduction:

- A high-FODMAP food from a different food category should be tested next, while the food group that the triggering food came from should be placed on a back burner, and no other food from that group should be tested until all other food groups have been tested.
- Later, the food group that triggered the sensitivity may be retested, ideally with a different food this time. The new food may

cause less sensitivity, and as time passes, the body's sensitivities can change.

Recommended FODMAP Challenge Foods

To effectively identify which food groups cause sensitivities, it is important to conduct the reintroduction challenge among foods that contain just one of the FODMAP sugars. One example is the fruit group's mango, which contains a large quantity of fructose. In another case, cow's milk, from the dairy food group, contains only one sugar, lactose. Testing foods like these ensure an accurate reading of other, similarly constructed foods in their group.

FODMAP challenge foods contain only one of the FODMAP sugar groups.

The following table provides a guide to the different sugars and the FODMAP foods they represent. One challenge food should be tested per group and tested in increasing quantities for three days.

Challenge Sugar	Testable Foods: 3 Day Servings. Test 1 per Group.
Fructans	Honey: 1 teaspoon up to 1 tablespoon Mango: ¼ medium-sized up to 1 full medium
Sucrose	Blackberries: 3 up to 12

	Avocado: ¼ up to ¾
	Apricot: ¾ fresh up to 2 small
Mannitol	Portobello mushroom: ¼ up to 1
	Sweet potato: 100g up to 200g
	Cauliflower: 20g up to 70g
Lactose	Cow's milk: 60ml up to 250ml
	Cow's milk yogurt: 50ml up to 200ml
Fructan (Grain)	Wheat bread: 1 slice up to 2 slices
	Wheat pasta: 50g up to 200g (cooked weight)
Fructan (Garlic)	Garlic: ¼ clove up to 1 clove
Fructan (Onion)	Leek: ¼ medium up to ½ (white and green sections)
	Onion: 1 tablespoon up to ½
Galactans/GOS	Canned chickpeas (rinsed): ¼ cup up to 1 cup
	Almonds: 15 up to 25
	Silken tofu: 3 tablespoons up to ¾ cup
Fructose + Sorbitol	Apple: ¼ up to one whole
	Pear: ¼ up to one whole

Source: *Journal of Gastroenterology and Hematology.* Re- challenging FODMAPs: the low FODMAP diet phase two. (2017).

Phase 3: Integration

Upon completion of the elimination and reintroduction phases, you will be knowledgeable about high and low-FODMAP foods, and capable of choosing when and how to begin, maintain, and conclude your own low-FODMAP diet. Once you actually complete the first and second phases, you can begin the third phase, which is called integration, because it brings together the low-FODMAP foods you need to continue with because of sensitivity to alternative high-FODMAP foods, and the high-FODMAP foods you have proven you can tolerate. You now have the resources to know all the high-FODMAP foods that have the potential to create your digestive disorders, and you will have tested food in groups and individually, to identify the foods you can safely eat, and the foods you now know to avoid.

An Evolving Process

Is already underway. As you progress through the reintroduction phase, the foods that you discover to be tolerable may continue to be consumed; so in effect, the integration phase will have already begun, overlapping the reintroduction of the different saccharide group foods. You will be continuing to add tolerable high-FODMAP foods every day, adding to those already tested and accepted.

Ideal diet plan. With that knowledge and the self-confidence it brings you, it is time to create your own ideal diet plan and strategy for how your diet may evolve. Perhaps of greatest importance, you have a wide range of choices that are favorable to you, and safe for your digestive health. You will be able to bring foods back into your diet in a controlled way, based on what you can handle, and further enhanced by the knowledge you are gaining about your overall physical and emotional health. Your diet is that important, and that influential over your health and well-being.

The objective now is to establish your own, personalized, ongoing FODMAP diet. When you (on your own, or with a doctor's or dietician's oversight) have identified all of the tolerances you can stay with and all of the triggers that cause symptoms, you may reintroduce all of the high-FODMAPs that are tolerable, and, at the same time, being aware that you will not be returning to the high-FODMAP foods that you have found to be intolerable. Of course, nothing needs to be permanent, and over time, you may retest certain foods that need to be avoided now, but in time can become less intolerable to your body.

Do Not Be Sidetracked

Healthy foods? Accept that foods you like, and foods that are generally recognized as healthy, and "good for you," may be among the high-FODMAPs that may not be tolerable for you to digest without triggering symptoms. An apple a day may be reputed anecdotally to keep the doctor away, but not if you are symptomatically sensitive to that high-FODMAP fruit.

What about gluten? While gluten may be found in wheat, rye, and spelt grain-based foods, like bread and pasta, gluten is not a FODMAP or a carbohydrate; it's a complex protein. While you may want to observe a gluten-free discipline, be aware that gluten is not a low-FODMAP food, and does not need to be removed from a low-FODMAP diet.

Not just low-FODMAPs. Your new FODMAP diet can be for the long haul; forever, perhaps, but it should not be an exclusively low-FODMAP diet. You may feel terrific after the phase 1 elimination stage, with all your digestive symptoms relieved, but it's not good to continue beyond six weeks, at most. You need to resume the high-FODMAP foods that you can tolerate to ensure good and complete nutrition. As long as foods are not causing symptoms, feel encouraged to add them back in. Do not imagine there is something "wrong" with high-FODMAP foods.

You are unique. What you can tolerate, and what you cannot, will not be the same for others, except, possibly, for a close relative, in cases where genetics play a role in making a person susceptible to IBS or IBD. Do not be tempted to emulate another person who says, "I used to have IBS, but after the FODMAP diet, I am allowed to enjoy apples." Just because that person can tolerate apples does not imply that you can. Conversely, you may not be sensitive to the fructan in wheat, while another person is highly sensitive. Follow your own custom FODMAP-tested dietary plan, and enjoy a stress-free, discomfort-free lifestyle.

Have confidence. The best way to know if food sensitivities are the cause of your digestive tract symptoms is by following the disciplines of the low-FODMAP diet. Estimates indicate that many people with IBS, IBD, or other food-induced digestive disorders can reduce or fully eliminate their symptoms by following the disciplines of the low-FODMAP diet and making the necessary adjustments: eliminating sensitivity-inducing high-FODMAP foods and returning tolerable high-FODMAP foods to their diet. You will enjoy eating while avoiding the risks of the symptoms returning, like gas and bloating, abdominal pain and cramps, and diarrhea or constipation.

On that note of enjoying eating, the following chapters are devoted to helping you not only survive the challenges of the elimination phase of the FODMAP diet but to make it as enjoyable and satisfying as possible.

Chapter 8:

Low-FODMAP Diet

Breakfasts

According to tradition, breakfast is the most important meal because it fuels you up for the physical challenges of the day. More recently, since most of us are not out in the fields farming all day, or exerting that much energy for as long, the statement has been called into question. Nutritionists acknowledge that breakfast is definitely important, and definitely not to be skipped, but its importance is equaled by lunch and dinner.

Breakfast means "breaking the fast," since the last meal may have ended 12 hours earlier, and yes, it is understandable that it's now time to recharge the body with carbohydrates, proteins, and fats. Our bodies need food for energy, and to build and rebuild our cells, organs, and muscles. Some of us wake up hungry and ready to eat, while others of us need some time to wake up and get going, and yet others of us prefer a workout before we dig in.

Whatever our personal preferences on the timing of breakfast, we all like to start the day with good tasting, nutritious foods, and you may be wondering if this is possible with the constraints of the low-FODMAP diet.

Rest assured that breakfast, and all other meals have been researched by dieticians and nutritionists to come up with quality options you will enjoy. Let's get cooking!

Low-FODMAP Meat and Cheese Bake

A rich, high protein hot and delicious loaf to enjoy at breakfast, especially on weekends, when you've slept a little later, woke up hungry, or when you are in the mood for a hearty breakfast that will hold you until lunch. Speaking of lunch, this recipe is well qualified to serve as a lunch option, or even shared with others during brunch.

Nutritional information per serving: 330 calories, 30 g carbohydrates, 16 g protein, 16 g total fat, 9 g saturated fat, 3 g fiber

Servings: 12

Prep Time: 20 minutes

Cook Time: 40 to 45 minutes

Ingredients:

- 24 oz ground beef, chicken, turkey, or pork
- 3 cups shredded or grated potatoes (peeled or unpeeled)
- 2 cups grated cheddar or Swiss cheese
- 1 cup Bisquick or other batter mix, gluten-free

- 2 cups lactose-free milk r nut-based milk substitute
- 4 eggs, medium or large
- ¼ tsp each of salt, pepper, oregano or thyme
- 1 tbsp extra virgin olive oil
- Cooking spray or vegetable shortening

Directions:

1. Preheat your oven to 400 F and place the rack in the center position.
2. Lubricate the rectangular pan with the cooking spray or shortening.
3. Brown the ground meat in the olive oil until fully cooked completely, or use leftover cooked ground beef.
4. Place the cooked meat in the baking dish.
5. Mix in the grated potatoes and half of the ground cheese to combine.
6. Mix well the eggs and milk then add in the Bisquick, and spices, and add on top of the meat, potatoes, and cheese mixture.
7. If this is being prepared in advance, cover with foil or plastic wrap and refrigerate.
8. When ready, put in the preheated oven for 40-45 min uncovered. Remove from the oven, cover with remaining cheese, and return to warm until the cheese melts.
9. Let stand 5 minutes, then serve.

Breakfast Corn Tortillas with Eggs

An easy-to-prepare tasty variation on lunch tortillas, with excellent nutritional values. Be sure to use corn instead of wheat tortillas to keep this low-FODMAP. Can be eaten at home, or packed to take with you. Add a few drops of lemon or lime juice to give a tart twist to the flavor notes.

Nutritional information per serving: 311 calories, 16 g carbohydrates, 20g protein, 17.3 g total fat, 7 g saturated fat, 4.7 g fiber

Servings: 4

Prep Time: 5 minutes

Cook Time: 10 minutes

Ingredients:

- 4 corn tortillas
- 4 eggs
- 2 tbsp macadamia dukkah
- ¼ tsp each salt and pepper, as needed
- 1 cup grated mozzarella
- ¼ cup lactose-free yogurt
- 4 diced medium-sized ripe tomatoes
- Parsley, cilantro, or other herb to garnish

Directions:
1. Boil the eggs in a medium pot for 5 ½ minute, remove and place under cold water to stop cooking. Peel when cool.
2. Heat the tortillas in a non-stick pan for 20 seconds on each side. Remove them to a covered container to keep them warm until all are heated.
3. Cover the tortillas with the yogurt, follow with the diced tomatoes and cheese.
4. Slice the eggs in half and place both halves of one egg on each tortilla. Sprinkle with herbs and dukkah, and salt and pepper, to taste.
5. The tortillas may be rolled and wrapped to take with you, if you're in a hurry.

Ham and Cheese Breakfast Bites with Spinach

This intensely satisfying breakfast selection has been kept low-FODMAP, yet it's nutritious, delicious, high in protein and beneficial fiber to satisfy the needs of your intestinal microbiota. This is a breakfast favorite that will keep you feeling full all morning. Pressed for time? Make this recipe in batches for freezing and have it ready when you are. Just pop it in the microwave, or take it with you to eat on the way.

Nutritional information per serving: 316 calories, 36 g carbohydrates, 17 g protein, 12 g total fat, 6.3 g saturated fat, 2.6 g fiber

Servings: 6

Prep Time: 10 minutes

Cook Time: 20 to 25 minutes

Ingredients:

- ½ cup oat bran or gluten-free oatmeal
- 1 ½ cup corn flour
- ½ tsp xanthan gum
- 2 ¼ tsp baking powder (to help rising)
- ⅓ cup lactose-free cream
- ½ to ¾ cup lactose-free milk - low fat
- 2 medium or large eggs
- 1 cup ham, diced, or torn into small pieces if sliced
- 1 ½ cup spinach, preferably baby leaves, sliced
- ½ cup chives, ½ tsp paprika, smoked, if available
- 1 cup cheddar cheese, grated or cubed
- Olive oil or spray to coat muffin pan

Directions:

1. Preheat your oven to 360 F.
2. Mix the flour, xanthan gum, and baking powder in a bowl.

3. **Separately, mix the eggs, milk, and cream, and then add the chives, ⅔ cup of the cheese, and ham.**
4. In the bowl with the dry ingredients, make a well (depression), and pour in the milk, cream, ham, cheese, and spinach mixture. Stir well to mix the wet and dry ingredients.
5. **Lightly coat the muffin pan with oil or spray, and pour in the mixture to almost, but not quite full. Sprinkle the remaining ⅓ cup cheese on each muffin. Add a pinch of paprika on top of each muffin.**
6. Bake until the cheese on top is golden brown, about 20 minutes.
7. Top with an herb sprig and a small sliver of tomato, if desired.

Crunchy Maple Granola

This is an updated improvement to traditional breakfast cereals, with more nutrients, and great flavor. Feel free to vary the ingredients with other low-FODMAP nuts, seeds, and dried fruits. This is a big recipe that will create 20 servings, and save you time on most days, but you can scale down to smaller, or even individual servings. Take a chunk with you, or break up a section, put in a bowl and add milk for a super crunchy cereal. Another idea: add cocoa powder or instant coffee to the mix to add some flavor. Stick to the suggested portion size to keep the fat level under control.

Nutritional information per serving: 178 calories, 12 g carbohydrates, 5 g protein, 12 g total fat, 4 g saturated fat, 3 g fiber

Servings: 18 to 20

Prep Time: 5 minutes

Cook Time: 20 minutes

Ingredients:

- 1 ½ cups rolled oats (oatmeal)
- ¼ cup flax seeds or linseeds
- ½ cup almonds
- ¼ cup each of sunflower and chia seeds
- ½ cup buckwheat kernels (groats)
- ¼ cups pepitas (pumpkin or squash seeds)
- ½ cup dried cranberries
- ½ tsp cinnamon (ground)
- ½ cup pure maple syrup
- ¼ cup coconut or olive oil
- 2 tsp extra virgin olive oil
- 30 g natural, pure peanut butter
- 1 tsp vanilla extract

Directions:
1. Line two pans with parchment paper, and preheat the oven to 360 F.
2. Chop the almonds, and then mix all dry ingredients in a bowl.

3. Put all wet/moist ingredients in a container you can safely microwave, and then heat until fully liquid, but do not overheat.
4. Add the liquid to the dry ingredients, and mix thoroughly, ensuring full coating.
5. Spoon the mixture onto the paper-lined pans in a thin coating, and press down
6. Sprinkle dried cranberries over the top of the mixture.
7. Cook for between 15 to 18 minutes, or until golden color. Remove to cool.
8. Once it's cool, break the granola in each tray into about 10 pieces, and store in an airtight container for up to four weeks.

Overnight Rich Oatmeal

Have you ever been in the mood for oatmeal for breakfast, but just didn't want to take the time and effort? It actually takes only five minutes to cook oatmeal (the regular type, not instant), but if that's not fast enough, try this easy-to-prepare version that you mix up the night before and refrigerate. Cooking time? None, unless you want to give the bowl one minute in the microwave before serving. Oatmeal has become a rockstar among foods because its fiber is credited with lots of health benefits, even preventing heart disease. With added dairy, this bowlful has quality protein, is low in saturated fat, and the fruit in this recipe gives it sweetness.

Nutritional information per serving: 368 calories, 38.5 g carbohydrates, 12 g protein, 16 g total fat, 3 g saturated fat, 5 g fiber

Servings: 2

Prep Time: 10 minutes

Cook Time: 0 minutes

Ingredients:

- 1 cup oatmeal (rolled oats)
- 16 to 20 almonds
- 2 tbsp dried cranberries
- 2 tbsp pepitas (pumpkin or squash seeds)
- 1 to 2 tsp cinnamon (ground)
- ½ cup lactose-free milk, or rice, almond, soy milk
- ½ cup water
- ½ banana, sliced, 4-6 strawberries ¼ cup blueberries
- 2 tbsp lactose-free yogurt
- 1 tsp maple syrup (pure), optional

Directions:

1. Pulse oats and almonds in a food processor or blender, and pulse a couple of times, to mix and make almond pieces smaller. Alternatively, roll a wine bottle or rolling pin over the almonds to crack them.

2. Mix oats, almonds, and other dry ingredients in a bowl.
3. Add the milk and water, (and maple syrup), cover, and refrigerate overnight.
4. In the morning, remove your half-serving and put it in a bowl. Add the fruit and yogurt on top, and mix or leave on top.
5. If you prefer to serve warm, heat for one minute in the microwave before adding yogurt.

Spinach Omelet with Feta and Pine Nuts

If a great-tasting, protein-rich breakfast is your priority, this low-FODMAP omelette will check all your boxes. The combination of eggs, feta cheese, pine nuts and spinach bring together a delicious dish that is both fast and easy to prepare. Be creative (if you want) and toss in shredded ham or other meat for even more protein and additional flavor.

Nutritional information per serving: 337 calories, 2.2 g carbohydrates, 24 g protein, 26 g total fat, 8.6 g saturated fat, 2.2 g fiber

Servings: 1

Prep Time: 5 minutes

Cook Time: 5 minutes

Ingredients:

- 2 large eggs

- i cup baby spinach leaves
- 1 tbsp lactose-free milk (or low-FODMAP alternative)
- ¼ cup feta cheese, crumbled or chopped into chunks
- ½ tsp butter
- 1 tbsp pine nuts, toasted, if available
- salt and pepper to taste

Directions:
1. Warm the spinach and feta in a lightly oiled pan until the leaves wilt, or heat together in the microwave for 20 to 30 seconds.
2. Add eggs and milk in a bowl and whisk with a fork until well blended, and eggs are fully mixed.
3. Use a frying pan or skillet to melt the butter over moderate to low heat.
4. Once the butter is melted and sizzling, pour the egg mixture into the pan, and tilt it so the egg mixture evenly covers the bottom of the pan.
5. Keeping the heat moderate, wait until the omelet starts to show firmness, then pour the feta and spinach mix on one-half of the omelet.
6. Sprinkle the pine nuts on top of the feta and spinach.
7. Tilt the pan and using a spatula, flip the side of the omelet without the mix over the side with the mix.

8. Allow the omelet to cook for another 30 seconds, then tilt the pan and slide the omelet onto your plate.
9. Sprinkle lightly with salt and pepper if desired, and serve with low-FODMAP bread, toasted.

Vegan-Style French Toast

If you are a vegan, and prefer not to eat animal-sourced foods, or if you are interested in adding vegan meals into your lifestyle, this recipe is for you. You can enjoy, without losing any of the good taste and nutrients we associate with French Toast. In France, this is known as "pain perdu," or lost bread, meaning it's a good way to use older bread that may be a bit stale, but otherwise a valuable part of any meal.

Nutritional information per serving: 335 calories, 28 g carbohydrates, 19 g protein, 14.4 g total fat, 1.6 g saturated fat, 3 g fiber

Servings: 1 portion

Prep Time: 5 minutes

Cook Time: 5 minutes

Ingredients:
- 2 slices of low-FODMAP bread: no wheat, rye, or spelt (but sourdough bread with these grains is okay)
- ⅓ cup tofu, soft version

- ¼ cup soy milk (made with soy protein)
- ¼ tsp vanilla extract
- 1 tsp olive oil or other vegetable oil for cooking (or cooking spray)
- Maple syrup (pure, natural) for serving
- Banana, berries, for topping (optional)

Directions:
1. Put the soy milk, tofu, and vanilla extract in a blender or food processor, and mix well, or place in a bowl and whisk thoroughly.
2. Pour the wet mixture into a flat pan or dish, and place the bread in the liquid to soak.
3. Turn the slices of bread so that both sides are coated, and the bread is saturated with the liquid.
4. Coat a non-stick frying pan or skillet with the oil or cooking spray, and place on a medium-high burner. As soon as the oil or spray is hot, place the slices of bread in the pan.
5. Cook for about two minutes, then check to see the progress by lifting the edge of a slice with a fork: if the slices are golden-brown, flip them over. If not, give them a bit more time.
6. When both sides are cooked, put the slices on a plate, and top with maple syrup, and berries, or sliced banana.

Porridge with Quinoa, Yogurt, and Banana

Porridge is frequently what the British, Australians, and New Zealanders call hot breakfast cereal, and it's often made with traditional grains, like oats or cream of wheat. But here we have an interesting low-FODMAP version, made with quinoa, which is a high protein grain originating in Bolivia and other parts of South America. Quinoa is one of the few grains that contain complete protein, with all the necessary amino acids our bodies need to build muscle. This recipe runs a little higher in calories due to the high protein (19 g) and carbohydrates (76 g), but it's low in fat and especially low in saturated fat.

Nutritional information per serving: 470 calories, 76 g carbohydrates, 19 g protein, 9 g total fat, 4.2 g saturated fat, 6.7 g fiber

Servings: 1

Prep Time: 5 minutes

Cook Time: 10 minutes

Ingredients:

- ½ cup quinoa flakes
- ½ cup lactose-free milk, soy milk made from soy protein
- ⅔ cup water
- ⅓ ripe banana
- ¼ cup lactose-free yogurt (or Greek yogurt if you can tolerate lactose)

- 1 tsp maple syrup (pure, natural)
- Cinnamon to sprinkle (optional)

Directions:
1. Pour the water and half the milk into a small pot or saucepan, and bring to a boil.
2. Add the quinoa flakes, mix, and turn down the heat to low.
3. Simmer the mixture for 5 or 6 minutes, and slice the banana, keep to the side.
4. When the quinoa flakes have absorbed all the liquid, remove from heat, and spoon or pour contents of the pot into a serving bowl.
5. Add the remaining milk, yogurt, and banana slices. Mix, and top with the maple syrup, and optional cinnamon for a flavor boost.

Chapter 9:

Low-FODMAP Diet Main Meals

We tend to take lunch and dinner, our main meals, with greater seriousness than breakfast, at least on one basis: we expect more variety in our main meals, and while we might have the same breakfast almost every day (or at least, every weekday), we vary our lunches, and especially, our dinners.

It's easy to fall into thinking that breakfast is boring, so to avoid repetition, hopefully the last chapter's breakfast recipe suggestions should encourage some experimentation. But now, we're onto the bigger show, and you will definitely see a diversity of choices for your lunches and dinners.

Chicken Cacciatore

This is a traditional favorite, deep in color, high in aromas, and outstanding in flavors, which mingle and fill the home with appetite-stimulating fragrances. The name means "hunter's style" chicken in Italian because it contains an array of seasonal ingredients that are available at the time of cooking; sort of a pot-luck situation, where whatever you have goes into the same pot. This recipe will feed a large family, or can serve to provide lots of leftover meals. It uses low-FODMAP ingredients and is easier to prepare than you may think.

Nutritional information per serving: 345 calories, 14 g carbohydrates, 27 g protein, 18 g total fat, 4.3 g saturated fat, 8 g fiber

Servings: 8

Prep Time: 10 minutes

Cook Time: 40 minutes

Ingredients:

- 6 chicken thighs, bone in, skin and fat removed
- 1 bunch scallions, green part only, chopped
- 4 tbsp extra virgin olive oil
- 2 large carrots
- 1 eggplant (aubergine), medium size
- 1 red bell pepper, seeds removed
- 1 celery root (celeriac), medium size, peeled
- 1 can (about 16 oz) diced tomatoes, Italian or domestic
- ½ cup pitted olives (like Kalamata), halved
- 1 cup oyster mushrooms, or canned (do not use fresh button or portobello)
- 1 cup chicken stock, or water
- 1 tsp oregano (dried)
- 1 tsp rosemary (dried), or 2 sprigs fresh

- 1 tsp sugar (optional)
- 1 tsp black pepper (cracked or ground) and 1 ½ tsp salt
- 1 cup fresh basil, parsley, or cilantro leaves

Directions:
1. Warm the olive oil in a large pot or saucepan.
2. When the oil is hot, add all vegetables (except the olives and mushrooms), plus the scallion greens, herbs, and spices.
3. Stir well, coating all ingredients with oil, and cook for 8 minutes, and then add the chicken thighs, olives, mushrooms, diced tomatoes, and stock or water, mixing well.
4. Preheat the oven to 360 F.
5. Carefully pour the contents of the pot into a large casserole that is oven safe.
6. Add the basil, parsley, or cilantro leaves.
7. Cover the casserole with a lid, or aluminum foil, and place in the oven on a mid level rack. Cook for 34 to 40 minutes. If sauce has not yet thickened, remove the covering and cook for another 10 minutes.
8. Serve with brown rice, or low-FODMAP pasta (made with rice or quinoa).

Salmon with Potato Chunks

One of the recommended sources of protein on heart-healthy diets (like the Mediterranean diet) is fish, and one of the most recommended fish is salmon, due to its high level of omega-3 antioxidants, along with the highest quality essential amino acids to form nutritionally complete protein. Plus, salmon tastes great, can be prepared in a number of ways, and is easy to make. Potatoes are a good companion to salmon, and these roasted chunks are ideal.

Nutritional information per serving: 391 calories, 26 g carbohydrates, 26.6 g protein, 20 g total fat, 5 g saturated fat, .23 g fiber

Servings: 4

Prep Time: 10 minutes

Cook Time: 60 to 65 minutes

Ingredients:

- 4 Atlantic, Scottish, or Norwegian salmon fillets, about ½ lb each
- 2 tsp extra virgin olive oil
- 8 to 10 small potatoes, skin on (to retain nutrients)
- Herbs (fresh or dried) to taste (optional), plus salt, to taste

Directions:
1. Scrub the potatoes to remove traces of soil, and place in a pot of boiling, lightly salted water. Cook for 20 minutes, and then remove to cool.
2. Preheat the oven to 430 F, and slice the potatoes into thick chunks or slices.
3. Scrape the sides of the potatoes with the tip of a fork to roughen the surface for better absorption and browning.
4. Line a wide tray with parchment paper (or aluminum foil), and arrange the salmon filets and potato chunks.
5. Sprinkle the olive oil over the salmon and potatoes, then turn over so oil is on all surfaces of salmon and potatoes; salmon should be skin side down for cooking.
6. Place the tray in the oven and bake for 20 to 25 minutes; there is no need to turn the salmon.
7. Remove from the oven and serve with a green seasonal salad.

Spicy Chicken Soup with Rice Ramen Noodles

A good, flavorful chicken soup is always a welcoming comfort food, but it's especially good to have when it's cold out, or when we're feeling under the weather. This version is high in nutrition, and with the added flavors that take it out of the ordinary, and fill the home with tempting, exotic fragrances. Unlike traditional chicken soup, which can take a full day to prepare and cook, this one takes 60 minutes from start to finish. Want even more nutrition? Add low-FODMAP vegetables, like carrots, celery, kale, spinach, and zucchini.

Nutritional information per serving: 178 calories, 12 g carbohydrates, 5 g protein, 12 g total fat, 4 g saturated fat, 3 g fiber

Servings: 2

Prep Time: 15 minutes

Cook Time: 45 minutes

Ingredients:

- 2 chicken breast fillets, small, skinless
- 2 tsp sesame oil, and 2 tsp olive oil (optional: garlic-infused)
- 2 tbsp soy sauce; 2 tsp minced ginger
- 1 ½ tbsp rice wine vinegar
- 2 tsp white (table) sugar
- 4 cups chicken stock (check label to ensure low-FODMAP ingredients)
- 1 bunch bok choy
- ½ cup finely chopped scallions, green part only
- 2 medium/large eggs
- 1 cup precooked rice (brown or white)
- Salt and pepper, as needed

Directions:

1. Preheat the oven to 375 F, and season the chicken breast fillets with salt and pepper.
2. Add the olive oil to an oven safe large pan, and place over medium heat.
3. Place the chicken fillets in the pan and cook until a golden-brown color, about 5 minutes on each side.
4. Place the pan with the chicken breasts in the oven for 15 minutes, to fully cook the chicken.
5. Carefully remove the pan from the oven, place the chicken on a plate, and cover with foil to keep warm.
6. In a large pot, heat the sesame oil, and then add the minced ginger until it softens, then add the rice wine vinegar, soy sauce, and sugar. Cook for another 1 to 2 minutes, then add the stock and bring to a slow boil.
7. Simmer the stock and other ingredients, uncovered, for 5 minutes then toss in the bok choy and continue to simmer for a few more minutes.
8. Separately, cook the eggs by immersing them in boiling water and simmering for 8 minutes. Be sure to retain the simmering water for the noodles, as you remove the eggs and run under cold water to cool and stop cooking.
9. When cool enough, peel the eggs, slice in half, lengthwise, and set aside.

10. Add the rice to the boiling water, and thinly slice the chicken breasts and set aside. Continue to boil for about 3 minutes.
11. Remove the rice from the water, drain, and divide between 2 bowls. Add the chicken slices and soup liquid to the bowls, and serve.

Brown Rice Pilaf with Vegetables and Herbs

Rice pilaf is a welcome comfort food that is easy to make with ingredients you can change up based on taste and what you have available (avoiding onions and garlic, which are high-FODMAP). Brown rice is recommended because it has all its bran fiber, vitamins, and minerals, which are polished off of white rice. You can enjoy this rice pilaf by itself for a lighter lunch, or make it into a heartier lunch or dinner by adding protein, like grilled beef, chicken, or fish. If you want to skip the grilling, consider adding dried beef (unseasoned), or smoked salmon. You can also open a can of tuna and mix in with the pilaf before serving. Vegetarians and vegans can add tofu, in regular, smoked, or grilled form.

Nutritional information per serving: 190 calories, 30 g carbohydrates, 4 g protein, 6.7 g total fat, 1.4 g saturated fat, 3 g fiber

Servings: 4

Prep Time: 20 minutes

Cook Time: 50 minutes

Ingredients:

- 2 cup brown, or basmati rice, uncooked
- 3 tbsp extra-virgin olive oil (optional: garlic-infused)
- 1 small zucchini, diced
- ½ red bell pepper
- ½ medium eggplant (aubergine), diced
- 3 tsp curry powder
- 1 tsp turmeric powder
- 2 ¾ cups beef, vegetable, or chicken stock (check label to avoid high-FODMAPs)
- 1 ½ tsp cracked or ground black pepper, plus salt to taste
- ⅓ cup chives, chopped
- ⅔ cup fresh basil leaves, chopped
- Lemon juice to serve (optional)
- Lactose-free yogurt, for serving (or Greek yogurt if you are lactose-okay)

Directions:

1. Heat the oil in a nonstick pot or saucepan that has a lid available for later, and after 1 minute, add the bell pepper, eggplant, and zucchini. Raise the heat, and saute for 4 to 5 minutes, or until they start to brown, stirring frequently so nothing sticks or burns.
2. Add the spices (not the chives or basil herbs), and stir well, and cook for 1 to 2 more minutes.

3. Add the rice, stir into the mix, and saute for 2 minutes.
4. Add the stock, stir well, and bring the liquid to a boil, then turn down heat, and simmer uncovered for 10 minutes.
5. Place the lid firmly on the pot, and continue to cook for 30 minutes, either over low heat on the cooktop burner, or (if the pot is ovenproof) in the oven preheated to 360 F.
6. Remove from the burner or oven after 30 minutes, and allow to rest with the lid on for 15 minutes.
7. Remove the lid, stir in the chives and basil, and top with lemon juice and yogurt to serve (optional).
8. If not serving four, refrigerate and save the leftovers.

Chicken and Potato Salad

A well-made chicken salad is a good choice for a light, low-FODMAPs lunch, and this one has chunks of potatoes,and added flavor from a mustard mayonnaise dressing. You can make it from scratch in the morning for lunch, or for greater ease, make it the night before, and keep it covered in the refrigerator. The lean chicken provides high protein and low fat, and all salad components are low-FODMAP. This salad is easily transportable, just be sure to store it in the refrigerator until ready to eat.

Nutritional information per serving: 256 calories, 20.5 g carbohydrates, 14 g protein, 13 g total fat, 2 g saturated fat, 4.4 g fiber

Servings: 4

Prep Time: 10 minutes

Cook Time: 20 minutes

Ingredients:

- 2 large or 3 medium skinless chicken breasts
- 2 medium potatoes
- 2 radishes, small
- 1 tbsp extra virgin olive oil
- 1 cucumber
- 2 tomatoes, medium size, firm
- 2 cups baby spinach leaves, packed
- 2 tsp mustard, wholegrain if available
- 4 tbsp mayonnaise

- 2 tsp lemon juice
- ½ tsp maple syrup (pure, natural)
- Salt and pepper, as desired

Directions:
1. Wash and dry the potatoes then chop into small chunks, and place in a pot or saucepan.
2. Cover the potatoes with water, and bring to a boil; reduce the heat and simmer for 15 minutes, then drain and allow to cool.
3. Using a sharp knife, slice the chicken breasts into bite-size pieces.
4. Mix the chicken pieces in a bowl with olive oil, and salt and pepper, as desired.
5. Heat a fry pan or skillet on medium-high, and once the pan is hot, pour in the chicken and stir, occasionally, for 5 minutes, or until the chicken is cooked through and golden in color. Remove from heat.
6. Wash and dry the radishes, tomatoes, and cucumber, then slice each into bite-size pieces.
7. Create your mustard mayo mix by blending the mustard, mayonnaise, lemon juice, and maple syrup in a cup or jar.
8. Prepare individual servings by spooning a small amount of mustard mayo onto the bottom of the serving bowls, followed by layers of each ingredient (spinach, cucumber, tomato, potato, chicken), then follow with another sequence of

mustard mayo and salad components. Save a small amount of the mustard mayo to pat on top.
9. Serve immediately, or refrigerate for later.

Tuna Salad Niçoise

This salad is a French favorite that can be made easily with short preparation time, and with available, healthy, low-FODMAP ingredients. The combination of tuna and eggs ensures high protein, and you'll be getting a high level of fiber that your intestinal microbiota will appreciate. (If you want even more fiber, swap brown rice or quinoa for the potatoes.) The fat content seems a bit high, but it's due to beneficial, heart-healthy olive oil.

Prepare this salad for a nutritious lunch, or a light dinner, either just before serving, or if you prefer, pop it in the refrigerator the evening before. Keep your tuna salad covered and cool until you're ready to dig in.

Nutritional information per serving: 550 calories, 34 g carbohydrates, 36 g protein, 28.7 g total fat, 5.4 g saturated fat, 8.8 g fiber

Servings: 1

Prep Time: 5 minutes

Cook Time: 20 minutes

Ingredients:

- 1 can tuna in olive oil
- 1 medium potato, boiled
- 1 cup butter lettuce leaves, cut into strips
- 6 cherry tomatoes, or 1 large tomato, cut in chunks
- Green beans (stringbeans), about 6 to 8 thick styles
- 1 hard-boiled egg, quartered lengthwise
- 4 to 6 pitted and halved green or black olives
- 1 anchovy filet, marinated in olive oil, drained and cut into pieces
- ½ tsp mustard
- 3 tsp rice wine vinegar

Directions:

1. Dice the potato, boil in water for 15 minutes, until tender, then drain and set aside.
2. Toss the green beans into the water and simmer for just 1 minute (they should be bright green at this point), then use a fork or slotted spoon to scoop them out, rinse under cold water to stop cooking, and set aside.
3. In a bowl, place the lettuce, string beans, anchovy, tuna (undrained, broken into chunks if it comes out of the can solid), olives, potatoes, and tomatoes. Add the mustard and vinegar, and toss all the ingredients to mix well. If there

was not enough olive oil in the tuna can, add another tsp to the mix.
4. Place the sliced egg on top, season with salt and pepper, and serve.

Skillet Ground Beef and Vegetables

You can make this hearty, filling, and nutritious stew quickly and easily, so even if you haven't planned anything, it can be on the table in 30 minutes. The eight ingredients provide a diversity of color, flavors, and textures, and make a low-FODMAP, low-carbohydrate meal.

Nutritional information per serving: 280 calories, 24 g carbohydrates, 22 g protein, 10 g total fat, 5 g saturated fat, 3 g fiber

Servings: 2

Prep Time: 10 minutes

Cook Time: 20 minutes

Ingredients:

- 1 tbsp avocado oil or extra virgin olive oil
- 2 medium carrots, chopped
- 3 medium florets of broccoli, chopped
- 2 large or 4 small radishes, chopped
- 1 small zucchini, chopped
- 1 small yellow squash, chopped

- ¾ lb ground lean beef, grass-fed if available
- 1 tsp ground ginger
- Salt and pepper for seasoning

Directions:
1. Take a medium or large skillet, cast-iron, if possible, and add the avocado or olive oil. Turn a burner on medium heat and heat the oil until it starts to smoke about 1 minute.
2. Add the chopped carrots, broccoli, and radishes, stir well, cook on medium heat for 1 minute, then lower the heat and cover. Allow to steam for 2 minutes.
3. Remove the cover, stir the vegetables, then use a spatula or wide spoon to push the vegetables to one side of the skillet.
4. Place the ground beef into the empty part of the skillet, and flatten with the spatula to fill the empty space, and turn the heat back up to high.
5. Season with salt and pepper, and after 1 minute, flip the ground beef over, and sprinkle with ground ginger, wait 1 minute to allow the meat to brown on the bottom side, then use the spatula or spoon to chop up the beef into small pieces and chunks.
6. Mix the ground beef with the vegetables, and stir for 1 minute, then add the chopped zucchini and yellow squash, and mix all ingredients.

7. Lower the heat, and cover, allow to steam and simmer for 10 minutes.
8. Uncover, mix well, allow to cook for 1 to 2 minutes, remove from heat and serve. Cover leftovers and refrigerate to reheat when needed.

Mediterranean-Style Salmon

With salmon being richly flavorful, high in quality complete protein, nutritiously loaded with antioxidants and healthy oils, easy to prepare in a variety of ways, and even being relatively inexpensive compared to many other types of fish, it's surprising that more people are not eating salmon more often. Maybe it's simply a lack of familiarity, with most of us raised on beef, lamb, chicken, and pork. You can broil or grill a salmon filet or steak anytime, in the oven or on the outdoor grill, but this more flavorful recipe can be made at home in the kitchen. The secret is using parchment paper to hold everything together during cooking, and preventing the scents and flavors from escaping. This is a low-FODMAP dish with all the essences and benefits of the Mediterranean diet.

You may vary the number of servings by allowing ½ lb salmon per person, and increasing the amounts of herbs and vegetables.

Nutritional information per serving: 320 calories, 20 g carbohydrates, 24 g protein, 16 g total fat, 6 g saturated fat, 4 g fiber

Servings: 2

Prep Time: 10 minutes

Cook Time: 30 minutes

Ingredients:

- 1 ½ lb salmon filet (Atlantic, Scottish, or Norwegian, preferably)
- ½ tsp salt
- ½ tsp paprika
- ½ tsp ground ginger
- ½ tsp dried dill plus 1 ½ tsp chopped fresh dill
- 6 to 8 Kalamata olives, chopped
- 2 tbsp stewed sun-dried tomatoes
- 2 artichoke hearts, sliced
- 1 tbsp capers
- 2 tbsp pesto sauce

Directions:

1. Preheat the oven to 400 F.
2. Place the salmon filet skin side down on a sheet of parchment paper.
3. Sprinkle the salt and paprika evenly over the filet, also add ginger and dried dill, then spoon on the olives, sun-dried tomatoes, artichoke hearts, capers, and pesto sauce.
4. Fold the parchment paper over the salmon filet, both ends first, then both sides; tie the sides lightly with string so the parchment paper

remains closed during cooking (it may be necessary to tie each end as well as the sides).
5. Carefully place the wrapped fish in a flat pan and place on a center rack in the oven.
6. Bake at 400 F for 20 minutes.
7. Remove the wrapped fish from the oven, and place on a counter.
8. Cut the strings, fold back the paper (being careful of escaping steam).
9. Using a sharp, large knife, cut the filet into serving pieces, and using a wide spatula, lift the slices onto the serving plates, being sure not to let the herbs and vegetables slip off.

Chapter 10:

Low-FODMAP Diet Desserts

Desserts on a low-FODMAP diet? Of course. Following the lists that designate the foods are safe to eat during the challenging elimination phases makes the challenges less formidable. Yes, some of your old favorites may have to wait until the FODMAP diet is in a second or third phase, and some desserts you look forward to may become altered to meet the low-FODMAP criteria.

You will be pleasantly surprised because serious cooks have come up with alternatives that not only meet the low-FODMAP lists but are downright terrific. After all, low-FODMAP foods include fruits and vegetables, almost all nuts and seeds, flavorful grains to replace wheat and rye, plus natural sweeteners, even sugar, and maple syrup. There will be no reason to be unhappy with any of these approved low-FODMAP recipes.

Almond Blueberry Muffins (Vegan friendly)

This is a simple recipe that is not only high on the taste scale, but is made without animal products—no eggs, no dairy—so vegetarians and vegans can enjoy it too. This recipe is for a dozen muffins, so take it easy if you want more than one or two, because the calories are high for the size, due to the oil content. Fortunately, saturated fats are very low.

Nutritional information per serving: 286 calories, 2 g carbohydrates, 2 g protein, 17.4 g total fat, 1.8 g saturated fat, 1 g fiber

Servings: 1

Prep Time: 25 minutes

Cook Time: 25 minutes

Ingredients:

- 2 cups gluten-free flour (a mix of 2 or more: rice, potato, tapioca, and quinoa flours)
- 1 tbsp chia seeds, boiled in 3 tbsp of water
- ½ cup almond meal (reserve 1 tbsp for sprinkling later)
- 1 tsp baking powder
- ½ cup sugar
- ⅔ cup vegetable oil
- 1 tsp vanilla extract
- ¾ cup almond milk
- 1 cup blueberries, fresh (preferably), or frozen

Directions:

1. Preheat the oven to 350 F, and insert paper cups to line a 12 muffin pan.
2. Boil the chia seeds in a small bowl, allow to thicken and swell for 15 minutes.
3. In a larger bowl, combine the flour, almond meal, sugar, and baking powder, mixing the dry ingredients well.
4. Add the liquids: almond milk, vegetable oil, vanilla extract, plus the chia seeds.
5. Stir the mixture until just fully combined, and add a bit more almond milk if the mixture is too thick.
6. Carefully mix in the blueberries, take care not to break too many as you mix.
7. **Fill ⅔ of each lined muffin cup with the mixture; if any mixture is left, you may add a bit more to each cup, but do not exceed ¾ cup capacity, and then sprinkle each muffin with a little of the reserved almond meal.**
8. Place the muffin pan in the oven for 25 to 30 minutes, and remove when muffins are lightly brown, and serve when cool. The remaining muffins can be frozen or stored in an airtight container.

Peanut Butter and Cacao Bowl

The harmonious relationship between peanut butter and chocolate has been well established, and this low-FODMAP version of the combination does not disappoint! You can prepare and have it ready in just a few minutes, so be sure to give it a try. Vegetarians and vegans can exchange the lactose-free milk with non-dairy alternatives.

Nutritional information per serving: 365 calories, 33 g carbohydrates, 12.45 g protein, 19 g total fat, 5.4 g saturated fat, 5.4 g fiber

Servings: 1

Prep Time: 5 minutes

Cook Time: 2 minutes

Ingredients:

- 1 tbsp peanut butter (pure, natural)
- 1 tsp cacao powder
- 1 banana (not too ripe)
- 1 tsp maple syrup (pure, natural)
- 1 tsp chia seeds
- ½ cup lactose-free milk, or non-dairy milk substitute (almond, soy)

Directions:

1. Put all ingredients in a blender or food processor, and blend for 20 to 30 seconds, and serve.
2. Peanuts or strawberries can be used as toppings, to add flavor, texture, and fiber.
3. If you don't have a blender, keep all ingredients at room temperature, place in a bowl, and stir vigorously until well mixed. Serve immediately or refrigerate to chill.

Pecan Pie

This time-tested favorite is usually associated with the Fall season, Thanksgiving, and the end of year holidays, but there's no reason why pecan pie can't be enjoyed year around. There are a few extra ingredients and steps compared to some of the other recipes, but worth the effort to prepare this low-FODMAP special dessert.

Nutritional information per serving: 614 calories, 58 g carbohydrates, 8 g protein, 40 g total fat, 12 g saturated fat, 2.5 g fiber

Servings: 8

Prep Time: 30 minutes

Cook Time: 60 minutes

Ingredients:

- 1 cup gluten-free flour (a mix of 2 or more: rice, potato, tapioca, and quinoa flours)
- 1 cup water
- 2 tsp salt
- 2 tbsp butter, chopped and cold
- 2 medium eggs
- ⅔ cup brown sugar
- 1 tbsp maple syrup
- ⅔ cup rice malt syrup
- 1 tsp vanilla extract
- 1 cup pecans
- ½ tsp xanthan gum
- Lactose-free whipped cream, to top at serving

Directions:

1. Combine water, salt, and butter in a pot or saucepan.
2. Add 2 tbsp flour, xanthan gum, and bring to a simmer, stirring well with a wooden spoon or ladle until mixture is thick; remove from heat and allow to cool.
3. When the liquid is cooled, whisk in 2 eggs, adding one at a time, until both eggs are fully blended.
4. Add ½ cup of flour, mix partially, then ladle out the mixture onto a counter and knead the dough until it turns shiny; then wrap the dough in clear wrap and refrigerate.

5. When the dough is fully chilled, remove it from the refrigerator, unwrap, and preheat the oven to 392 F.
6. Roll the dough on a floured surface with a rolling pin (a wine bottle can substitute), until it is ½ cm thick, or about ¼ to ⅓ inch.
7. Gently lift the pastry and place in a buttered, loose bottom fluted pie dish (or, any low-sided pie pan will suffice), and press down with fingertips. Trim the edges.
8. In a saucepan or small pot, cook the rice malt, butter, sugar, and maple syrup over low heat, stirring until butter is melted and the mixture is smooth.
9. Remove the pot from the heat, and allow to cool slightly; whisk in 2 more eggs, the vanilla, and stir well.
10. Spread the pecans over the pastry, evenly, then pour the syrup over the pecans
11. Reduce oven heat to 350 F, and place pie on an oven tray and bake for 35 minutes, or until dough is browned and firm.

Acai and Fruit Bowls

Here is an easy way to have your acai berries and not have to worry if high-FODMAPs have crept into your dessert, because thesssss recipe has been focused entirely on low-FODMAP ingredients.

Nutritional information per serving: 410 calories, 42 g carbohydrates, 12.4 g protein, 22 g total fat, 8 g saturated fat, 15.5 g fiber

Servings: 1

Prep Time: 5 minutes

Cook Time: 0 minutes

Ingredients:

- 15 raspberries
- 1 cup strawberries, stems removed
- ½ cup baby spinach leaves
- 2 tbsp acai powder (not containing inulin)
- ½ cup lactose-free milk or substitute (almond milk)
- 1 tsp maple syrup (pure, natural) (optional)
- ½ ripe banana, sliced
- ½ kiwi fruit, peeled, sliced
- 1 tsp dried (desiccated) coconut
- 1 tsp hemp seeds or chia seeds
- 1 tsp peanut butter (pure, natural) (optional)

Directions:

1. Put raspberries, strawberries, acai powder, spinach, milk, and maple syrup in a blender or food processor, and blend, adding the milk slowly to obtain the best consistency.
2. Pour into a bowl, and top with kiwi, banana, coconut, seeds, and peanut butter.

Banana Bread

This low-FODMAP version of a favorite fruit-based dessert cake can be prepared in just 10 minutes.

Nutritional information per serving: 225 calories, 31 g carbohydrates, 2.9 g protein, 10.2 g total fat, 1.7 g fiber

Servings: 12

Prep Time: 10 minutes

Cook Time: 60 minutes

Ingredients:
- 3 medium ripe bananas, mashed
- ⅓ cup coconut oil
- 2 large eggs
- ½ cup maple syrup (pure, natural)
- 1 tsp vanilla extract
- ¼ cup almond milk (unsweetened)
- 1 tsp baking soda
- 1 cup gluten-free flour
- ½ tsp ground cinnamon
- ½ tsp salt
- ½ cup chopped walnuts

Directions:
1. Preheat the oven to 325 F, and line a bread loaf pan with parchment paper edges reaching above the sides of the pan.

2. Briskly mix the oil and maple syrup in a medium-size bowl, then add the eggs and whisk, and then whisk in the mashed bananas, almond milk, and vanilla extract.
3. Add and mix the baking soda, gluten-free flour, salt, and cinnamon in a large bowl. Follow with the wet ingredients and stir well until all ingredients are mixed, and then stir in the chopped walnuts. This is your batter.
4. Pour the banana bread batter into the loaf pan, and bake for 60 minutes. Remove from the oven, and allow your low-FODMAP banana bread to cool before lifting the parchment paper to remove the banana bread from the pan.
5. Slice and serve.

Peanut Butter Brownie Truffles (No-bake!)

When a scrumptious bite-size combination of peanut butter and chocolate plus healthy fiber-loaded oats can be made without baking, it's almost impossible to resist giving it a try. How can anything that tastes this good be so good for you, and strictly low-FODMAP? Good for a quick dessert, or anytime you're in the mood for a succulent snack that will give you an immediate energy boost.

Nutritional information per serving (1 ball): 96 calories, 11 g carbohydrates, 3 g protein, 4.2 g total fat, 2 g fiber

Servings: 18

Prep Time: 10 minutes

Cook Time: 0 minutes

Ingredients:

- 1 cup oatmeal (rolled oats, regular, not precooked)
- ½ cup peanut butter (pure, nothing added)
- ¼ cup chocolate chips (don't use milk chocolate)
- 2 tbsp cocoa powder
- ¼ cup maple syrup (pure, natural)
- 2 tbsp chia seeds
- ¼ tsp salt (optional)

Directions:

1. Pulse the oats and peanut butter in a blender or food processor until well mixed (if you don't have a blender or processor, do all the mixing in a bowl using a large spoon, and be sure the peanut butter is room temperature because it will be too hard to mix if cold).
2. Mix in the chocolate chips, cocoa powder, maple syrup, chia seeds, and salt.
3. Pulse or mix with the spoon until well mixed, and if the mixture seems too dry, add a tbsp of maple syrup or more until the right consistency—slightly sticky, and easy to roll—is achieved.

4. With clean hands, form a 1-inch-sized ball, by taking a chunk of the mixture and rolling it into a round shape (it doesn't have to be perfect; lop-sided or oval shapes still taste great!).
5. Place the ball on a pan that you have lined with parchment paper, or wax paper, and continue with the remaining mixture (you may also place the balls directly onto a non-stick pan or skillet).
6. Place the tray or pan in the freezer until the balls are no longer sticky, and then put them in a container for storage.
7. The balls may be stored in the refrigerator, or in the freezer, if you don't mind waiting for them to thaw before you enjoy them.

Chocolate Cream Pie

A classic, a favorite, a delight to have for dessert, yet it's easy to make, with only 10 minutes of prep time, and as long as you keep it to a single serving, it's low-FODMAP (so resist the temptation; your gut and your waistline will thank you).

Nutritional information per serving: 260 calories, 35 g carbohydrates, 3.6 g protein, 12 g total fat, 8 g saturated fat, 0.4 g fiber

Servings: 10

Prep Time: 10 minutes

Cook Time: 1 hour 15 minutes

Ingredients:

- 6 large egg whites
- 6 tsp sugar
- 4 tbsp cacao powder plus 2 tsp in reserve to sprinkle
- ¼ cup, grated dark chocolate
- ½ to ⅔ cup whipped lactose-free cream for topping
- 1 tsp balsamic vinegar

Directions:

1. Preheat the oven to 356 F, and separate the egg yolks and whites; reserve and refrigerate the yolks for later use.
2. Beat the egg whites, until the liquid stiffens and peaks form, then add the sugar, 1 tsp at a time, while you continue to beat, and the mixture remains stiff and shiny.
3. Mix in the cocoa powder, vinegar, and grated dark chocolate, but mix lightly, not aggressively.
4. Place a sheet of parchment paper (or other grease-proof paper) in a baking tray or ovenproof flat pan, and pour and spoon out the mixture onto the paper, to form a circle shape, about 10 inches/24 cm in diameter.
5. Smooth the sides and top of the mixture, using the bottom of a large spoon, and then place the

tray or pan in the oven, and immediately turn down the heat to 300 F.
6. Bake for 1 ¼ hours, then turn off the oven, and leave the door open, allowing your chocolate cream pie to cool, then remove and spread whipped cream over the top, then lightly sprinkle reserved cocoa powder.
7. You may add dark chocolate shavings, or low-FODMAP berries, as toppings.

Frozen Fruit Yogurt

For cold refreshment on a warm day, or evening, this easy to prepare frozen yogurt is a low calorie, low-FODMAP treat. The recipe calls for frozen strawberries and other fruits, so this frozen dessert can be served immediately. But you can benefit from what's available seasonally, and use fresh fruit, as long as you then freeze the mixture before it's served.

Nutritional Information per serving: 104 calories, 14 g carbohydrates, 6 g protein, 2.3 g total fat, 1.4 g saturated fat, 4 g fiber

Servings: 4

Prep Time: 5 minutes

Cook Time: 0 minutes

Ingredients:
- 1 cup (or ½ lb) strawberries, frozen

- 1 cup (or ½ lb) blueberries or raspberries, frozen (or other low-FODMAP berries)
- 1 tbsp sugar or maple syrup (optional, for added sweetness)
- 1 cup lactose-free yogurt (or Greek yogurt if you are lactose-okay)
- 1 tsp vanilla essence

Directions:

1. Put all ingredients into a blender or food processor, and blend until the mixture is smooth and creamy in consistency.
2. Spoon or scoop into bowls and serve immediately, or put in a container and place in the freezer for at least 1 hour (but then allow 10 minutes out of the freezer, to soften before serving).
3. Fresh fruit may be substituted for frozen fruit, but freeze the mixture, for serving later.

Chapter 11:

Low-FODMAP Diet

Snacks

When is a good time for a snack? When breakfast has worn off, and lunch is still far away? If lunch was light, or dinner is going to be late? What about late at night, just before bed when you're craving something sweet?

It seems like savory snacks, or on the saltier side, are good to have between meals, while sweet snacks fit when a little more energy is needed, or for a little treat at night. But there are no rules, so enjoy what you want, when you want, as long as you follow the low-FODMAP requirements, and all of these recipes do.

Banana Hazelnut Biscuits

These tasty hazelnut and seed biscuits are loaded with healthy oils and microbiome-loving fiber, yet have that touch of sweetness to keep you coming back for more. Just 5 minutes of preparation, and 12 minutes later you will be happily sampling your accomplishment, and feeling pretty good.

Nutritional information per serving: 153 calories, 9 g carbohydrates, 4 g protein, 10 g total fat, 3 g saturated fat, 3 g fiber

Servings: 12

Prep Time: 5 minutes

Cook Time: 12 minutes

Ingredients:

- ½ cup hazelnuts, chopped
- 1 banana, medium size, ripe
- 2 dates (dried), diced
- ¼ cup sunflower seeds (shelled), or linseeds
- 2 ½ cups peanut butter (pure, natural, no additives)
- 1 ½ cups chia seeds
- 1 tsp vanilla essence
- ¼ cup each: cranberries, oatmeal, desiccated coconut

Directions:

1. Preheat the oven to 356 F, and put all the ingredients in a bowl to mix well, making sure the banana is well mashed and mixed with other ingredients.
2. Line a baking pan or other flat, wide pan with parchment paper.
3. Spoon the mixture into 12 round balls and place each on the parchment paper.

4. Press down on each ball with the back of a spoon to achieve a flatter muffin shape.
5. Put the tray in the oven and bake for 12 minutes, or until they are golden.
6. Biscuits may be stored for several days in a ziplock bag or airtight container.
7. Feel free to try different low-FODMAP seeds and nuts.

Green Fruity Veggie Smoothie

It's cold, it's smooth, it's built-up with pineapple, spinach, and fiber-loaded chia seeds, plus protein-rich dairy (or alternatives), and it's ready in about 5 minutes. Snack on this smoothie anytime you feel the need for some refreshment, nourishment or energy.

Nutritional information per serving: 199 calories, 15.g carbohydrates, 7.6 g protein, 10.3 g total fat, 6 g saturated fat, 8 g fiber

Servings: 1

Prep Time: 5 minutes

Cook Time: 0 minutes

Ingredients:
- ⅔ cup fresh pineapple, chopped and placed in freezer for 5 minutes
- 1 cup baby spinach leaves

- ⅓ cup lactose-free milk, or soy protein milk or almond milk or hemp milk
- ¼ cup yogurt, lactose-free, or Greek if you are lactose tolerant
- 2 tsp chia seeds
- 1 ⅓ tbsp shredded coconut
- 4 to 6 ice cubes

Directions:
1. Put the chilled pineapple, baby spinach, yogurt, milk, chia seeds and the shredded coconut in a blender or food processor, and then place the ice cubes on top, and replace the cover.
2. Blend until the mixture is fully mixed and creamy in consistency (if it appears too thick, or won't blend smoothly, slowly add more milk).
3. Your smoothie is ready to serve and enjoy.

Crispy Kale Chips

These surprisingly nutritional and fun to eat snacker chips are made with kale, the super-veggie, which brings vitamins A, C, and K, plus manganese and bone-building calcium. One serving is only 68 calories, with almost no carbs and a couple of grams of protein. Preparation is just 5 minutes, and the whole job is done in 12 to 15 minutes, providing four servings of irresistible bite-sized chips that leave potato chips behind, while staying within the low-FODMAP guidelines.

Nutritional information per serving: 68 calories, 1.5 g carbohydrates, 2.2 g protein, 5.7 g total fat, 1.4 g saturated fat, 1.5 g fiber

Servings: 4

Prep Time: 5 minutes

Cook Time: 15 minutes

Ingredients:

- 1 bunch kale, preferably Tuscan (lacinato)
- 2 ½ tbsp finely grated pecorino romano or parmesan cheese (or a mix of both); use fresh cheese only, and do not use dried or dehydrated cheese
- 1 ⅓ tbsp extra virgin olive oil
- Salt and pepper, to season

Directions:

1. Preheat your oven to 320 F, and line two baking trays with parchment paper.
2. Separate the kale leaves from stems, and tear the leaves into small pieces, about 1 to 2 inches across, and then wash the pieces and pat dry.
3. Mix the kale leaf pieces, cheese, and olive oil in a bowl, and then arrange the pieces on the parchment paper (don't let the leaves overlap).
4. Bake for 12 to 15 minutes; kale leaves should be crisp.

5. Remove from the oven, sprinkle with salt and pepper, and you're ready to snack.

Spicy Molasses Cookies

Everyone likes cookies, and those on a low-FODMAP diet don't have to miss out! These easy to make and bake crispy cookies have a rich molasses flavor that is highlighted by the spicy tang of cinnamon, nutmeg, and ginger. The molasses is just enough to keep the cookies low-FODMAP, while providing minerals like iron and magnesium, plus B vitamins. If you would like a variation with more nutrients and fiber, switch one cup of flour for one cup of oatmeal. The oatmeal will make the cookies chewy, too.

Nutritional information per serving: 114 calories, 17 g carbohydrates, 0.4 g protein, 5 g total fat, 1 g saturated fat, 0.1 g fiber

Servings: 30

Prep Time: 15 minutes + 60 minutes for refrigeration of the dough

Cook Time: 10 minutes

Ingredients:

- 2 cups gluten-free flour: rice, potato, quinoa (not wheat, rye, or spelt)
- 1 egg, medium or large
- 1 cup sugar

- ¾ cup butter or margarine
- ¼ cup molasses
- 2 tsp baking powder
- ½ tsp ground nutmeg
- ½ tsp ground ginger
- 1 tsp ground cinnamon
- ½ tsp salt

Directions:
1. Melt the butter in a small bowl or cup in the microwave, and then put in a large bowl, and add the egg and sugar and mix until it becomes smooth. Add the molasses, baking powder, flour, cinnamon, ginger, nutmeg, and salt, and stir until the mixture becomes dough.
2. Cover the dough with plastic wrap and leave in the refrigerator for 1 hour; the dough should become firm.
3. Preheat the oven to 356 F, and spread parchment paper to cover a large oven proof tray or large pan.
4. Place the tray in the oven and bake for 10 minutes. The tops of the cookies should begin to crack.
5. Allow the cookies to cool for a couple of minutes before moving them to a wire rack for additional cooling (the wire rack allows the bottoms of the cookies to crisp; on a hard surface the bottoms may stay soft).

Veggie Rice Slice

This healthy, high protein, low carbohydrate snack is made with beneficial grains and vegetables, and is tasty enough to satisfy every snacking urge, whether it's late morning or mid-afternoon, or anytime. Brown rice is recommended because the outer husk contains B vitamins, minerals, unsaturated oils, and fiber to help your digestive flow and keep your microbiome satiated (white rice has its outer husk polished off). This recipe calls for zucchini and carrots, but you can use broccoli, celery, red, yellow, or green pepper, or any colorful vegetables you prefer. Prepare in advance to have it ready to enjoy hot or cold.

Nutritional information per serving: 206 calories, 8 g carbohydrates, 12 g protein, 14 g total fat, 6.8 g saturated fat, 2 g fiber

Servings: 4

Prep Time: 5 minutes

Cook Time: 55 minutes

Ingredients:

- ⅓ cup brown rice
- 1 medium zucchini, finely chopped or grated
- 1 small carrot, finely chopped or grated
- 3 eggs, lightly beaten
- ¾ cup cheddar cheese, finely chopped or grated

Directions:
1. Preheat the oven to 356 F, and line a mid-size loaf or baking pan with parchment paper allowing the paper to extend above the top of the pan.
2. **Precook the rice by boiling it in ⅔ cup water for 10 minutes, then remove from the heat and allow it to stand for 3 minutes.**
3. Pour the rice (and any remaining water) into a large bowl, and add the zucchini, carrot, eggs, and ½ cup of the cheddar cheese; stir to thoroughly mix all the ingredients.
4. Spoon the ingredients into the loaf pan, and top with the remaining ¼ cup of cheddar cheese.
5. Bake for 30 to 35 minutes until golden brown, then remove from the oven to cool.
6. Carefully pull up on the parchment paper to lift the loaf out of the pan; once it has cooled, you may slice the loaf into 4 slices.
7. Store in an airtight container and refrigerate. Enjoy it cold, or warm from the microwave.

Avocado and Egg Salad Sandwich

A sandwich makes a great snack, as long it is made with nutritious ingredients. It will keep you away from the vending machines and the junk foods and satisfy any between meal hunger pangs you may start to feel. If a full sandwich is too much for a snack, just cut the ingredients in two and make it a half-sandwich, share it with a friend, or save a half for later (just be sure to refrigerate).

Nutritional information per serving: 392 calories, 22 g carbohydrates, 28 g protein, 22 g total fat, 6 g saturated fat, 3 g fiber

Servings: 1

Prep Time: 10 minutes

Cook Time: 0 minutes

Ingredients:

- ½ medium avocado, ripe (soft to touch)
- 2 hard boiled eggs
- 2 tbsp lactose-free yogurt, (Greek or Icelandic if lactose tolerant)
- ¼ to ⅓ cup kale leaves, loosely packed
- 2 slices, wholegrain gluten-free bread (no wheat, rye, or spelt), toasted
- Salt and pepper to season

Directions:
1. Remove the peel and mash the avocado in a bowl.
2. Add the eggs and mash into the avocado.
3. Mix in the yogurt, add salt and pepper as desired.

4. Layer the mixture and the kale leaves between the slices of toasted bread.
5. Cut the sandwich in half, and enjoy one part, or both.

Cheesy Salad Sticks

Whether it's just a snack for you, or if you're sharing with friends, family, or guests, you'll be pleased with these low calorie, yet protein rich salad and bacon snacks on a skewer. Make as many as you want, and keep them in the refrigerator. The recipe includes blue cheese, which some people may find too tangy or salty, so feel free to use any cheese that's firm enough to stay on the skewer. The bacon is optional, and vegetarians can use tofu, but if you're okay with bacon, avoid the processed, chemical-loaded version, and look for a natural, minimally processed kind. Another option is turkey bacon, but again, go for one that is minimally processed.

Nutritional information per serving: 63 calories, 1.4 g carbohydrates, 6.6 g protein, 3.2 g total fat, 1.3 g saturated fat, 1 g fiber

Servings: 12

Prep Time: 15 minutes

Cook Time: 5 minutes

Ingredients:

- ½ iceberg or romaine lettuce
- 4 slices bacon or turkey bacon, natural preferably
- 12 small squares cherry tomatoes, red or mixed colors
- 12 squares blue cheese, goat, cheddar, or feta
- 12 wooden skewers, soaked overnight to avoid splintering

Dip:

- ¼ cucumber, finely chopped
- ½ cup lactose-free yogurt (or Greek, low fat, if lactose is okay)
- ½ tsp lemon juice
- ½ tsp fresh dill, finely sliced
- Blue cheese, crumbled (optional)

Directions:

1. Cook the bacon or turkey bacon slices and set aside to cool, then divide the 4 slices into thirds to make 12 pieces.
2. Cut the lettuce into 12 chunks, or wedges.
3. Thread each skewer with a wedge of lettuce, one piece of bacon folded in half, one cherry tomato, and finish with 1 cheese square.
4. Prepare the dressing by mixing well, in a medium size bowl, the chopped cucumber, yogurt, lemon juice, sliced dill, and crumbled blue cheese (optional), salt and pepper to taste.

5. Keep the bowl of dressing handy for the skewers to be dipped.

Cheese and Herb Polenta Bites

Polenta is an Italian-syle grain that is actually ground corn. You'll see it on the shelf as cornmeal or coarse ground cornmeal. The taste of this polenta is enhanced when it's roasted, and especially when blended with herbs and cheese. There's no meat, so this recipe is okay for vegetarians. You have a choice of herbs and cheeses to use, and can use a mix, if you wish.

Nutritional information per serving: 178 calories, 12 g carbohydrates, 5 g protein, 12 g total fat, 4 g saturated fat, 3 g fiber

Servings: 4

Prep Time: 10 minutes + 4 hours (or overnight) to solidify

Cook Time: 30 minutes

Ingredients:
- 1 cup cornmeal polenta (dried, uncooked)
- 1 tbsp fresh, chopped rosemary, oregano, sage, or thyme
- ½ cup grated pecorino romano or parmesan cheese (or preferred cheese)
- Olive oil spray (or 1 tsp olive oil)

Directions:
1. Cook the polenta in water or low-FODMAP vegetable stock, according to package directions, and grease the inside surfaces of a flat baking tray, using olive oil spray, or wipe with a small quantity of olive oil.
2. When the polenta is thick and creamy, mix in the grated cheese and herbs, stir well, and then remove from heat and pour into the baking tray.
3. Cover the tray with plastic wrap, and chill in the refrigerator for 4 hours, or preferably overnight.
4. Remove the tray and invert (flip) over a counter or large chopping board, and tap to let the polenta fall onto the counter or board.
5. Slice the polenta into small triangular, square, or rectangular shapes (use a butter knife or spatula to protect the counter).
6. Preheat the oven to 460 F, and line a baking tray with parchment paper, and spray with olive oil, or wipe with a small quantity of olive oil, using a cloth or paper towel (do not soak the paper; just a very light coating of oil or spray).
7. Place the polenta bites on the tray, making sure pieces are separate, and bake for 20 minutes, or until pieces are golden-brown.
8. Remove from the oven, and sprinkle with some grated cheese and chopped herbs, or fresh basil leaves, and add cherry tomatoes, if desired.

Conclusion

My objective in writing this book has been to educate you on the importance of having a healthy gastrointestinal system, help you understand how it works, how it can become dysfunctional, and cause painful, disruptive symptoms. While some gut disturbances may be inherited, most conditions we are aware of are due to imbalances caused by the diet, and specific foods that cannot be digested normally. We have identified these dietary disruptors, and covered the FODMAP diet to bring a range of debilitating symptoms under control.

This has been an expedition into the human digestive system from one end to the other, as we follow the food we eat on its incredible journey from ingestion, to digestion, assimilation, and finally, elimination.

Along the way you have discovered the vast population of bacteria and viruses that inhabit your gastrointestinal tract, especially in the small and large intestines, where most of their beneficial action takes place. These trillions of microbes, collectively called your microbiome, aid the digestive process, and keep essential hormones in balance, by maintaining a conversation with your brain to inform it of conditions. Your life-protecting immune system is strengthened when your microbiome is in balance.

You nourish and sustain your microbiological partners with the foods you eat, especially the fiber you've been encouraged to increase in your diet, with whole grains, complex carbohydrates like fruits and vegetables, plus nuts and seeds.

But not all your microbes are beneficial: other, less positively-oriented bacteria and viruses may find their way into the microbiota, and wreak havoc if allowed to run amok. Here's where disorders like irritable bowel syndrome (IBS), inflammatory bowel disease (IBD), and its best known conditions, Crohn's disease, and ulcerative colitis, create serious symptoms that can disrupt a lifestyle. If this isn't enough, the bad bacteria can weaken the small intestinal walls, letting toxins and bacteria pass into the bloodstream, a condition called "leaky gut."

Fortunately, researchers in Australia and the UK have discovered the probable cause, FODMAPs, short for Fermentable Oligosaccharides, Disaccharides, Monosaccharides, And Polyols, which are short chain carbohydrate molecules found in many foods, and which some of us cannot digest properly. In those cases, these saccharides and polyols find their way into the large intestine, where malevolent bacteria feast on them, generating toxins and hydrogen gas, and leading to the chronic cramps and excess gas, stomach pain, diarrhea, and constipation, that are the symptoms of IBS and IBD. Leaky gut may also be a consequence of this negative bacterial action.

By removing all high-FODMAP foods from your diet during a brief elimination phase, it is possible for you to not only stop the serious gastrointestinal disturbances, but to gradually reintroduce these foods, one saccharide group at a time, to identify which high-FODMAP foods you can handle, and which you can't. Therefore, the low-FODMAP diet is not forever: at the conclusion of the elimination, reintroduction, and integration phases, many high-FODMAP foods may be back in your diet, and your long-term dietary directions can be established. You may even retest foods you can't tolerate every six months, or so, to see if your intolerance continues, or has lifted.

You Can Do This!

If you, or someone you know, suffers the symptoms of IBS, IBD, leaky gut, or any other serious GI tract disturbances, the FODMAP diet might just be the answer. Everything you need to know, is outlined for you, or for whomever you are counseling. Be optimistic, knowing that the challenging elimination phase lasts for only several weeks, and during this time, the low-FODMAP recipes will surely see you through.

If you have thoroughly benefitted from reading this book, and believe that others who suffer from digestive system disorders could benefit as well, please consider giving this book a favorable review on Amazon. This will send a signal to other potential readers who need help, and will reassure them that this book is for them.

I trust you will experience excellent health and well-being on the long road of life that lies before you, and wish you my very best. Thank you for letting me share my knowledge with you.

Reference List

American Heart Association. (2020). Healthy living - saturated fat. https://www.heart.org/en/healthy-living/healthy-eating/eat-smart/fats/saturated-fats

Aryal, S. (2020, June 9). The human digestive system - organs, functions, and diagrams. *Microbe Notes*. https://microbenotes.com/the-human-digestive-system-organs-and-functions/

Bell, B. (2017, February 2). Is leaky gut syndrome a real condition? An unbiased look. *Healthline*. https://www.healthline.com/nutrition/is-leaky-gut-real

Biology Online. (2020). Monosaccharide. https://www.biologyonline.com/dictionary/monosaccharide

Biology Dictionary. (2019, October 4). Disaccharide. https://biologydictionary.net/disaccharide/

Biology Online. (2020). Oligosaccharide. https://www.biologyonline.com/dictionary/oligosaccharide

Bourassa, L. (2019, October 4). Pros and cons of the low-FODMAP diet. *Verywell Fit*.

https://www.verywellfit.com/low-fodmap-diet-pros-and-cons-4705955

Brusie, C. (2020, March 6). Crohn's disease medications and treatments. *Healthline*. https://www.healthline.com/health/crohns-disease/medications

Cafasso, J. (2020, July 7). What does it mean to have chronic constipation? *Healthline*. https://www.healthline.com/health/cic/what-does-it-mean

Campos, M. (2017, September 22). Leaky gut: what it is, and what does it mean for you? *Harvard Health Publishing*. https://www.health.harvard.edu/blog/leaky-gut-what-is-it-and-what-does-it-mean-for-you-2017092212451

CBS News. (2012, July 31.). Gluten-free diet fad: are celiac disease rates actually rising? https://www.cbsnews.com/news/gluten-free-diet-fad-are-celiac-disease-rates-actually-rising/

CDC. (2020). What is viral hepatitis? https://www.cdc.gov/hepatitis/abc/index.htm

CDHF. (2020). Phases of the FODMAP diet explained. https://cdhf.ca/health-lifestyle/phases-of-the-fodmap-diet-explained/

Crohn's & Colitis. (2020). Never let Crohn's or UC keep you down. https://www.crohnsandcolitis.com/

Davis, N. (2018, March 26.) The human microbiome: why our microbes could be key to our health. *The Guardian.* https://www.theguardian.com/news/2018/mar/26/the-human-microbiome-why-our-microbes-could-be-key-to-our-health

Diet vs. Disease. (2018, November 21). Your complete guide to polyols and health. https://www.dietvsdisease.org/what-are-polyols/

Dr. Herbert's Team. (2020). Top 17 list of foods contain prebiotics. *Dr. Health Benefits.* https://drhealthbenefits.com/pharmacy/probiotic/foods-contain-probiotics-naturally

Enders, G. (2017, November). The surprisingly charming science of your gut. *TED.* https://www.ted.com/speakers/giulia_enders

Epicured. (2020). The low FODMAP diet and food list. https://mmm.epicured.com/low-fodmap-food-list

Eske, J. (2019, August 21). What to know about leaky gut syndrome. *Medical News Today.* https://www.medicalnewstoday.com/articles/326117

Evans. What you should about H-2 blockers for acid reflux. https://evens.com/learn/acid-reflux-treatments/h2-blockers-acid-reflux-treatment

Everyday Nutrition. (2020). Irritable bowel syndrome & low FODMAP diet. https://everydaynutrition.com.au/irritable-bowel-syndrome-low-fodmap-diet/

FODMAP Everyday. (2020). Low FODMAP diet. https://www.fodmapeveryday.com/ibs-fodmaps/low-fodmap-diet/

Fody Foods. (2020). Understanding each phase of a low FODMAP diet. https://www.fodyfoods.com/pages/understanding-each-phase-of-a-low-fodmap-diet

Foster, J. (2020, September 1). 6 FODMAP diets for IBS + who could benefit. *Self Hacked.* https://selfhacked.com/blog/fodmap-diet/

Gohil, K, and Carramusa, B. (2014, August). Ulcerative Colitis and Crohn's disease. *Pharmacy & Therapeutics.* https://www.ncbi.nlm.nih.gov/pmc/articles/PMC4123809/

Gunnars, K. (2018, November 9). FODMAP 101: a detailed beginner's guide. *Healthline.* https://www.healthline.com/nutrition/fodmaps-101

Harvard Health Publishing. (2011, April). Proton-pump inhibitors. https://www.health.harvard.edu/diseases-and-conditions/proton-pump-inhibitors

Harvard Health Publishing. (2011, March). What to do about gallstones. https://www.health.harvard.edu/womens-health/what-to-do-about-gallstones

Harvard T.H. Chan School of Public Health. (2020). The microbiome. https://www.hsph.harvard.edu/nutritionsource/microbiome/

Huzar, T. 2018, November 22). What is the difference between IBS and IBD? *Medical News Today*. https://www.medicalnewstoday.com/articles/323778

IBS Diets. (2020, October 22). FODMAP food list. https://www.ibsdiets.org/fodmap-diet/fodmap-food-list/

Jacoby, S. (2019, March 19). Leaky gut syndrome isn't an official diagnosis, but the symptoms are real. *SELF*. https://www.self.com/story/leaky-gut-syndrome

Julia. (2020). 40 low FODMAP dinner recipes. *The Roasted ROOT*. https://www.theroastedroot.net/40-low-fodmap-dinner-recipes/

Julie. (2020). Ultimate step-by-step guide to the FODMAP elimination phase. *Calm Belly Kitchen*. https://calmbellykitchen.com/blog/step-by-step-guide-to-the-fodmap-elimination-phase

Kubala, J. (2018, January 25). The 8 most common food intolerances. *Healthline*. https://www.healthline.com/nutrition/common-food-intolerances

Macon, B.L. (2019, March 22). Understanding gallstones: type, pain, and more. *Healthline*. https://www.healthline.com/health/gallstones

Marsh, A., et al. (2015, May 17). Does a diet low in FODMAPs reduce symptoms associated with functional gastrointestinal disorders? A comprehensive systematic review and meta-analysis. *National Library of Medicine*. https://pubmed.ncbi.nlm.nih.gov/25982757/

Mayo Clinic. (2020). Celiac disease. https://www.mayoclinic.org/diseases-conditions/celiac-disease/diagnosis-treatment/drc-20352225

Mayo Clinic. (2020). Crohn's disease. https://www.mayoclinic.org/diseases-conditions/crohns-disease/symptoms-causes/syc-20353304

Mayo Clinic. (2020). Gastroesophageal reflux disease (GERD). https://www.mayoclinic.org/diseases-conditions/gerd/symptoms-causes/syc-20361940

Mayo Clinic. (2020). Hepatitis C. https://www.mayoclinic.org/diseases-conditions/hepatitis-c/diagnosis-treatment/drc-20354284

Mayo Clinic. (2020). Irritable bowel syndrome. https://www.mayoclinic.org/diseases-conditions/irritable-bowel-syndrome/symptoms-causes/syc-20360016

McMillen, M. (2013, August 14). Leaky gut syndrome: what is it? *WebMD*. https://www.webmd.com/digestive-disorders/features/leaky-gut-syndrome%231#1

Monash University. (2020). High and low FODMAP foods. https://www.monashfodmap.com/about-fodmap-and-ibs/high-and-low-fodmap-foods/

Monash University. (2020). Recipes. Monash low FODMAP recipe index. https://www.monashfodmap.com/recipe/monash-low-fodmap-recipe-index/

NIH. (2020). Your digestive system and how it works. https://www.niddk.nih.gov/health-information/digestive-diseases/digestive-system-how-it-works

Raman, R. (2019, October 29). The leaky gut diet plan: what to eat, what to avoid. *Healthline*. https://www.healthline.com/nutrition/leaky-gut-diet

Robertson, R. (2017, June 17). Why the gut microbiome is crucial for your health. *Healthline*.

https://www.healthline.com/nutrition/gut-microbiome-and-health

Rossi, M. (2017, February 13). 10 foods that are high in FODMAPs (and what to eat instead). *Healthline.* https://www.healthline.com/nutrition/foods-high-in-fodmaps

Scarlota, K. (2020). Low FODMAP diet checklist. *Square Space.* https://static1.squarespace.com/static/53ced146e4b0ffc87f7fe427/t/5f2b0bf2c2671124c8715680/1596656627890/Low+FODMAP+Checklist+2020_tab.pdf

Schwartz, E. (2020). Easy low FODMAP recipes. *Fun without FODMAPs.* https://funwithoutfodmaps.com

Scott, A. (2017, August 28). Getting started on the low FODMAP diet: elimination phase. *A Little Bit Yummy.* https://alittlebityummy.com/getting-started-on-the-low-fodmap-diet-elimination-phase/

Scott, A. (2015, May 24). Getting enough fiber on the low FODMAP diet. *A Little Bit Yummy.* https://alittlebityummy.com/getting-enough-fibre-on-the-low-fodmap-diet/

The Free Dictionary. (2020). Bile. https://medical-dictionary.thefreedictionary.com/bile

Tuck, C., Barrett, J. (2017, February 28). Challenging FODMAPs: the low FODMAP diet phase two.

Journal of Gastroenterology and Hepatology. https://onlinelibrary.wiley.com/doi/full/10.1111/jgh.13687

Walker, W.A. (2020). Faculty and research directory. *Harvard T.H. Chan School of Public Health.* https://www.hsph.harvard.edu/w-walker/

Watzke, H. (2010, July). The brain in your gut. *TED Global.* https://www.ted.com/talks/heribert_watzke_the_brain_in_your_gut

WebMD. (2020, October 19). Natural treatments for Crohn's disease. https://www.webmd.com/ibd-crohns-disease/crohns-disease/ss/slideshow-crohns-natural-treatments?ecd=wnl_spr_112820&ctr=wnl-spr-112820_nsl-Bodymodule_Position2&mb=MukfT6opS3AxbF5kSEwI0ng0WleHxvIqssh%40W36l9r4%3d

WebMD. (2020, February 9). FODMAP diet for Crohn's disease. https://www.webmd.com/ibd-crohns-disease/crohns-disease/ss/slideshow-ibd-fodmap-diet

WebMD. (2020). Digestive disorders: prebiotics. https://www.webmd.com/digestive-disorders/prebiotics-overview

WebMD. (2020). Foods that fight GERD. https://www.webmd.com/heartburn-gerd/ss/slideshow-foods-fight-gerd

WebMD. (2020). Your digestive system. https://www.webmd.com/heartburn-gerd/your-digestive-system%231#1

Wikibooks. (2020). Fundamentals of human nutrition - you are what you eat. https://en.wikibooks.org/wiki/Fundamentals_of_Human_Nutrition/You_Are_What_You_Eat

Yawitz, K. (2019, October 17). Low FODMAP food list: what can you eat on a low FODMAP diet? *Diet vs. Disease.* https://www.dietvsdisease.org/fodmap-food-list/